When Blood Breaks Down

When Blood Breaks Down

Life Lessons from Leukemia

Mikkael A. Sekeres

The MIT Press

Cambridge, Massachusetts | London, England

This book was set in ITC Stone Serif Std and ITC Stone Sans Std by Toppan Best-set Premedia Limited. Printed and bound in the United States of America.

Library of Congress Cataloging-in-Publication Data

Names: Sekeres, Mikkael A., author.
Title: When blood breaks down : life lessons from leukemia / Mikkael A.
  Sekeres.
Description: Cambridge, Massachusetts : The MIT Press, [2020] | Includes
  bibliographical references and index.
Identifiers: LCCN 2019025810| ISBN 9780262043724 (hardcover) | ISBN
  9780262357814 (ebook)
Subjects: | MESH: Leukemia—psychology | Patients—psychology |
  Physician-Patient Relations
Classification: LCC RC643 | NLM WH 250 | DDC 616.99/4190019—dc23
LC record available at https://lccn.loc.gov/2019025810

10   9   8   7   6   5   4   3   2   1

To my wife, Jennifer, and children, Gabriel, Samantha, and Silas, for their unwavering love and support, and for always reminding me what really matters; for my parents, brother, and teachers, I still need your guidance; and always, always for my patients, who inspire me every single day.

Contents

Acknowledgments

This is perhaps the most difficult section of the book to write, as there is a half-century full of people to thank for the experiences that went into its creation.

First, my mentors: Brian Strom, MD, MPH, who taught me in medical school how to think critically and how to conduct clinical research; Stephanie Lee, MD, MPH, who honed these skills during my fellowship and clued me in on the right questions to ask; Richard Stone, MD, who patiently (so patiently) took my skull full of mush and filled it with knowledge of how to treat people with leukemia, and to do so with dignity, humanity, and even humor; Ilene Galinsky, MSN, ANP, and Barbara Tripp, RN, CNS, who did the same, and still do the same; and Brian Bolwell, MD, and Matt Kalaycio, MD, who continue to lead by example with caring and empathy.

Next, my friends: Doug Neu, Noam Neusner, and Shoshana Landow, MD, MPH, my oldest and dearest, who have been steadfastly supportive for decades; David Steensma, MD, Timothy Gilligan, MD, Hetty Carraway, MD, MBA, Nate Pennell, MD, Alison Loren, MD, and Jay Baruch,

MD, my mid-life friends, colleagues, writing buddies, and the people I turn to when my writing and research insecurities rear their ugly heads; Karl Theil, MD, for the images and, you know, for everything; and Jaroslaw Maciejewski, MD, PhD, my brilliant, closest research collaborator.

I am grateful to Caroline and Aaron Gerds, MD, MS, and Madeline Waldron, PharmD, who read versions of this manuscript and gave me such careful feedback, and helped ensure the accuracy of the stories and medical facts.

Toby Bilanow and Roberta Zeff, my editors at the *New York Times*, have been for years so encouraging, and so exquisitely skilled at transforming my essays into readable stories—their gentle guidance has been a gift.

My indefatigable agent, John Thornton of The Spieler Agency, believed in me from the moment he read a sample of this book in its first draft, and talked me off the ledge of despair more times than I care to admit! By offering his calm guidance and wise perspective, I believe he has qualified for an honorary degree in psychology.

Robert Prior, my editor at the MIT Press, also believed in me from the very beginning. His ability to mold text into something understandable, with great insight, has been extraordinary. What a pleasure to work so closely with someone like Bob. I am also grateful to Mary Bagg for her skilled copyediting, which put so many sentences back on the rails.

My wife, Jennifer, and my kids, were infinitely patient on car and plane trips while I remained undistracted and "in the moment" as I wrote this book, sometimes to their despair! You are my world, the loves of my life. And I don't care if that sounds cringey.

And finally, all of my patients, hundreds and hundreds of you, have taught me how to live a life, and to do so with such grace.

Preface

"Leukemia needs a better press agent."

I received this advice from my best friend when I told him what specialty I had settled on, soon after I had completed medical school. And in many ways, he was right. Leukemia has a terrible reputation. Before they even get to see me, many of my patients are told that their prognosis is grim and death is imminent. The word is so dreaded that no one in my own family spoke it louder than a whisper, fearing that to do so would somehow invoke the disease. What a wasted precaution: two family members developed leukemia anyway.

People are both terrified and fascinated by leukemia in all its forms. It is a monster—a malignant golem—that grows out of control and invades the organs within our own bodies. It is metastatic at its genesis.

Multiple times throughout the year, newspapers, television, and popular websites carry stories about possible causes of leukemias (mouthwash? baby powder?), the genetics of these diseases, what we can do to prevent them, and the newest therapies that might just (finally!) cure them. From

2017 to 2018, nine new drugs were approved by the FDA to treat leukemia, many of which take advantage of leukemia's own machinery to be its undoing.

The drama of the moment in which you are told you have leukemia can't be overstated. The world stops spinning. Priorities shift. Your brain can't function. Your rawest emotions, your worst fears, are laid bare, and yet somehow you have to regain your footing enough to make decisions about treatment and to define a new normal; if not for yourself, then for your partner and children.

Those who go into a remission from their leukemia, and who may even be cured, are granted a new lease on life, and often find they cherish the people and moments they previously took for granted. Those who fight leukemia for months or even years may somehow gather the strength, after all treatments have failed them, to decide that enough is enough, and spend their final hours living out what they should have been doing in their final decades.

Easily one-third of the medical residents who apply to our hematology-oncology fellowship program at Cleveland Clinic, in which they train to be cancer doctors—300 applicants for 6 positions per year—write an essay about a leukemia patient they cared for.

Why? Because there is that moment, when a doctor hears about a person whose blood counts are 10 or 20 or even 30 times higher than normal and wonders, "Am I going to be able to fix this?"

And then there's the next moment, when the patient meets this doctor who is supposed to solve the awful puzzle of a bone marrow gone horribly wrong. Together they move forward, one step after the other, developing a plan. Their lives become intimately entwined for months on end as the puzzle pieces are reassembled, the bone marrow functions normally again, and their plan turned out to be the right one.

Moments like these are precious in medicine. Heck, they are precious in life.

That's what drew me in.

When Blood Breaks Down tells the stories of three patients who arrive at the hospital, each within a day of the others.

Three people, all told to get their affairs in order when a blood test returned drastically wrong: Joan, a 48-year-old surgical nurse and mother; David, a 68-year-old husband, father, and grandfather; and Sarah, a 36-year-old pregnant mother and wife. One randomly thought, 24 hours earlier, that she was catching a bad cold; one that he was getting older and slowing down; one that she was exhausted from morning sickness.

And each one made decisions that no person should ever have to make: decisions that affect their lives, and the lives of those closest to them.

The three patients portrayed in this book are actually composites of people I have cared for over the years. The conversations, the medical twists and turns, the aspects of their lives that precede and follow their diagnoses all really occurred, though not necessarily to or for the persons to whom they are attributed. The discoveries that led to the treatment options for Joan, David, and Sarah, whose names

I chose as aliases, as well as the biologic basis of their cancers, are remarkable. So too is the research behind the causes of leukemia, how doctors and patients communicate with each other, and how we all handle a person whose death is imminent.

Perhaps most remarkable, though, is their undaunted spirit, their utter humanity in the face of a treasonous bone marrow that has turned on them.

The chance to have even a glancing relationship with inspiring people like this—that's what really drew me in.

MAS

1
Leukemia Arrives by Dark of Night

I jumped up and shook hands with this man who'd just given me
something no one else on earth had ever given me
I may have even thanked him habit being so strong
        —Raymond Carver, "What the Doctor Said," 1989

Joan Walker was a surgical nurse in Wooster, Ohio, near Amish country, who couldn't understand why she had become so tired every day, almost falling asleep on her feet while assisting doctors in the operating room.

"It felt like someone stuck a huge syringe into me and sucked out the energy, leaving me more tired than tired. I was a shell of a body, going through the motions of the day," she later told me.

Wooster, located about 50 miles south of Cleveland in Wayne County, is typical of the state of Ohio in many ways. It is headquarters to businesses such as Daisy Brand, the maker of sour cream and cottage cheese, and the Wooster Brush Company, which manufactures paintbrushes and rollers. It is also an agricultural center that encourages its young residents to participate in 4-H programs and compete at the Wayne County Fair.[1] As a result, industrial complexes and rural roads leading through bucolic farmland exist in equal measure. The patients Joan cared for reflected this balance, which she loved. Many, including Joan, had never left Wooster; their families, like hers, had lived in the area for generations and collectively pitched in to help raise the children. At the hospital, she often cared for her friends, and there were few secrets.

Perhaps it was years of waking up at 5 a.m. so she could be at the hospital on time for the first surgical case. Or the toll it took on her, being the single mom of two—a son who barely made it through high school and a difficult teenage daughter. It wasn't just the tiredness: her gums started to bleed every time she brushed her teeth, and she developed a rash on her legs under the compression stockings surgical nurses wear to combat the swelling that comes with hours of standing in the operating room. When she mentioned these symptoms to the doctor she had worked with for more than a decade, he insisted she have her blood counts checked.

Early on a Wednesday morning, after the first surgical case of the day, she went to the hospital's lab. With the technician who drew her blood, she joked about his ability to collect it on the first stick (he succeeded). After she had assisted on the second case of the day—a young man undergoing a hernia repair—the surgeon asked her to come into his office. He had just received a terrifying phone call from the lab.

Joan sat in a chair by the wall, still wearing her avocado-green scrubs. The surgeon sat in the chair behind his worn desk. Pictures of his wife and children adorned the walls, as did a photo of him with his surgical team, including Joan, taken a few years ago. She was still married back then, and was wearing her wedding ring.

She noticed his hair was mussed from the surgical caps he had been wearing all morning, and he made no effort to fix it. "Joan," he said to her, "your tests came back, and they were pretty abnormal." He grimaced and shook his head, clasping his hands in his lap as he leaned toward her. "I've never seen a white blood cell count this high. I need to get you over to someone who can figure out what's going on."

"How high?" she asked, looking her colleague in the eyes. Their professional relationship as doctor and nurse suddenly shifted; now, as doctor and patient, an unfamiliar vulnerability came into play for Joan, as it so often does when a healthcare worker gets sick.

"It's 154,000." They both knew that was over 15 times higher than normal. She swallowed the news and nodded her understanding.

"Do what you have to do," she told him.

He picked up the phone, called the hospital operator at the Cleveland Clinic, the hospital where I work, and for the first time, she heard someone use the word *leukemia* when referring to her. The operator paged me, and I broke from rounds to answer her summons. That was the first time I heard about Joan.

I took out a blank 3×5 card from the pocket of my white coat and jotted down some notes: "48 yr old fem . . . 4 wks of fatigue . . . gum bld . . . wbc 150k . . . hgb 7.3 . . . plt 18." The shorthand of illness. She was profoundly anemic, with a hemoglobin level that was about half normal, and her platelet count was one-tenth of where it should be, hence the bleeding.

"Yes, of course we'll accept her to the leukemia service," I told her doctor. He asked when she should leave for our hospital. "Today. If she would go home and pack her things and ask someone to drive her, that would be great." He assured me that she would do that. We said our goodbyes, and I returned to continue my hospital rounds, anticipating her arrival sometime that afternoon.

Few cancers can be considered "good" cancers, but acute leukemia is worse than most. Whereas more common cancers, such as those involving the breast or prostate, can take years to grow to a size that can be detected, acute leukemia develops quickly, over just a few weeks, and thus cannot be screened for. Also, unlike those solid tumors in which cancer cells lump into a mass (it is estimated that it takes 10 billion cancer cells to form 1 cubic centimeter of tissue, the size detectable on a CT scan considered to be abnormal), leukemia is a "liquid" tumor, filling the bone marrow space as it grows out of control.

The first description of leukemia has been attributed to a French surgical anatomist, Dr. Alfred Velpeau, in 1827. He wrote about "a florist and seller of lemonade, 'who had abandoned himself to the abuse of spirituous liquor and of women, without, however, becoming syphilitic.'" The patient had severe abdominal swelling, fever, headaches, and weakness, with an enormous liver and spleen, and pus-filled blood," as he described it, "like gruel."[2]

Despite Dr. Velpeau's insinuations, "sin" does not actually cause the cancer.

Leukemia was first classified as a distinct medical entity in 1845. The British pathologist Dr. John Bennett described it in an autopsy report on a 28-year-old slater from Edinburgh. Six weeks later, in early 1846, Dr. Rudolf Virchow, a prolific German pathologist who wrote more than 2,000 scientific papers and books, reported it in an autopsy he had performed on a 50-year-old female cook with an excessive number of white blood cells. Virchow named the condition *leukamie* in 1847, combining the Greek words *leukos* (white) with *aima* (blood). He was also the first to conclude that cancer arose from otherwise normal cells and that inflammation played a role.[3] There wouldn't be even a marginally effective treatment for leukemia, though, for another century.

Leukemia cells proliferate in an unfettered fashion, making too many primitive, nonfunctional white blood cells while the normal bone marrow cells that make the red blood cells and platelets die out completely. Those leukemia cells get packed so tightly in the bone marrow, eventually filling almost 100 percent of the bone marrow space, that sometimes they can't even be aspirated (sucked out) by one of our 4-inch-long, wide-bored bone marrow needles.

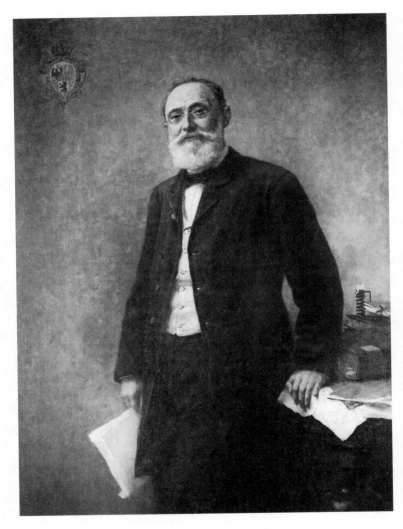

Figure 1.1
Dr. Rudolf Virchow, the pathologist who named leukemia. Portrait by Hugo Vogel, 1861.

What results is a paradox of sorts: too many cells in the bone marrow but too few cells in the blood stream—except for the white blood cells, whose numbers may be sky-high.

Leukemia is also in some ways more insidious than other cancers in that the symptoms are subtle until they suddenly become life threatening. Normally, the white blood cell count is between 4,000 and 11,000 cells per microliter of fluid, the hemoglobin (a measure of the red blood cells) is between 11.5 and 15.5 grams per deciliter of fluid, and the platelets are between 150,000 and 400,000 cells per microliter of fluid. With the death of the normal bone marrow cells, the resulting low red-blood-cell count, or anemia—in Joan's case a hemoglobin reading of 7.3 g/dL—causes people to feel tired, sleep more, and lose their appetite. The low platelets (18,000/µL for Joan) may cause minor bleeding from the gums or nose, or major bleeding leading to serious consequences, like a stroke, at lower levels. The high white-blood-cell count (154,000/µL for Joan), which can also occur with infections like the flu (though not nearly to as extreme a level as Joan's), can cause fevers and chills. That is, in fact, what most people think they have—a bad case of the flu that doesn't seem to go away.

That's what Joan thought she had.

Imagine the shock when someone with acute leukemia goes to her doctor, or an urgent-care center, thinking she has the flu, and a doctor walks into the exam room and tells her no, she has leukemia, and must be admitted to the hospital immediately for treatment. It's particularly daunting when that hospital is one of the largest in the world, almost 10 times the size of the hospital in Joan's community, with almost 1,500 hospital beds, 225,000 hospital admissions each year, and over 6 million outpatient visits.[4]

Imagine the shock when I walk into that person's room, trailed by a team that includes a hematology/oncology fellow, internal medicine residents, nurse practitioners, floor nurses, pharmacists, and students, and tell her that she needs to start chemotherapy within 24 hours, and may not survive the hospitalization. I would meet Joan later that day to have just that sort of conversation.

My team was waiting for me when I returned from answering the page.

"Sorry about that. Who's our next patient?" I asked.

Two interns and two second-year (or "junior") residents were standing in the hallway, each with a "workstation on wheels" (WOW), a laptop computer bolted to a platform that could be rolled from room to room. We document and store our patients' medical records electronically, so we use the WOW to write daily progress notes, record vital signs, order medications, and request consultations from specialists. (These workstations used to be called "computers on wheels" or COWs. But rumor has it that one day a patient on the gastric-bypass surgery floor overheard a nurse refer to her COW and mistakenly concluded that he was the subject of her conversation. He took offense, and the name was changed.)

The interns, both guys, were dressed sharply in pressed white shirts and thin ties, while the two junior residents were in various states of bedraggled, the most extreme example being John, who had a two-day growth of beard and stained hospital scrubs. He was post-call, having just spent the night caring for our patients and admitting new ones. At least his counterpart, Becky, was wearing clean scrubs.

I could fool myself into thinking that the interns and residents loved learning how to treat people with leukemia as much as I did, but for many this rotation was akin to being sentenced to hard labor in the Gulag. Rumors about the leukemia service ran rampant—that rounds can last until late in the day (what I called "continuous infusion" rounding, like chemotherapy that is administered as a constant drip over a 24-hour period); that the patients could get desperately ill and commonly needed to be transferred to the intensive care unit; and that the emotional toll, from caring for people who seemed fine one day but could be on death's door the next, was high.

All of that was true. But most interns and residents truly dreaded it because, despite the years they have spent in medical school learning about the science of disease and how we treat it, they still feared cancer. For some, it reminded them of their own family members who had cancer, endured toxic therapies, and still died. For others, they couldn't shake the popular misconception that a cancer diagnosis was tantamount to a death sentence.

Many also resented that I peppered them with inquiries during rounds. I not only quizzed them about disease-specific data, but also asked them for details about their patients, which at first blush seemed to have little to do with leukemia.

What types of inquiries elicited such resentment, you might wonder?

First were the questions anyone might expect me to ask while teaching trainees about medical conditions they would soon be treating: the typical clinical presentation and how to make a diagnosis of leukemia; what causes leukemia and how to treat it; the population incidence and prevalence of the disease; and how to estimate prognosis. And then there were those other questions, the ones that focused on the stories about people who have just arrived at our hospital. John started to speak.

"Mr. Sweeney is a 68-year-old man with a history of hypertension and kidney stones who was in his usual state of health until two months ago, when he started experiencing fatigue and shortness of breath when climbing stairs. He went to his primary-care doctor, who sent him for an EKG and pulmonary-function tests, both of which were normal. She then ordered labs, which showed pancytopenia." All of Mr. Sweeney's blood counts—the red and white blood cells and platelets—were low.

"What were the exact numbers?" I asked.

"He had a hemoglobin of 8.2, platelet count of 73,000, and white blood cell count of 1.8."

"Are you surprised that the white blood cell count was so low?" I followed up.

He thought about it for a few seconds. "No, because most older patients have a leukemia that probably evolved from another bone marrow problem."

"That's right." I commended him. He smiled. "How do you know that he has leukemia based on those blood counts, though?" I asked.

"I don't. But his primary-care doctor sent him to a hematologist, after scoping his GI tract to make sure he wasn't anemic from a GI bleed. That was normal. The hematologist performed a bone marrow biopsy, and it showed leukemia."

"What kind?" I inquired.

I was trying to get John to distinguish between the two acute forms of leukemia (acute myeloid leukemia, or AML, and acute lymphocytic leukemia, ALL) and the two chronic forms (chronic myeloid leukemia, CML, and chronic lymphocytic leukemia, CLL). Unlike acute leukemia, chronic leukemia can take years to develop and tends to be less life threatening—at first. Myeloid cells and lymphocytes are the two major branches of the immune system, with myeloid cells fighting bacterial infections, and lymphocytes fighting viruses. Table 1.1 includes basic facts about the different types of leukemia.

"It was AML," John said, handing me a copy of the pathology report. I read portions of it aloud to the team:

- "80 percent cellularity"—at his age, that should have been closer to 35 percent, or as a general rule, roughly 100 minus the patient's age

- "background of dysplasia"—as the resident indicated, this leukemia probably arose from a previous bone marrow cancer called myelodysplastic syndromes, in which the bone marrow cells are *dysplastic* (bad growing)

- "42 percent myeloblasts"

Table 1.1
The Different Types of Leukemia[5]

Type of Leukemia	Description	Number of Yearly Diagnoses (US, estimated)	Median Age at Diagnosis (years)	Treatment	Five-Year Survival
Acute Myeloid Leukemia (AML)	Cancer of the myeloid cells in the bone marrow; cells grow uncontrollably (proliferate) and stop maturing (*blasts*—comprising 20% or more of the bone marrow).	21,000	68	Intensive chemotherapy or Lower-dose chemotherapy or Watchful waiting Bone marrow transplant for high-risk AML or for relapse	30% (higher for good-risk features

Table 1.1 (continued)

Type of Leukemia	Description	Number of Yearly Diagnoses (US, estimated)	Median Age at Diagnosis (years)	Treatment	Five-Year Survival
Acute Promyelocytic Leukemia (APL)	Subtype of AML in which the cells stop maturing at the "promyelocyte" stage.	1,000	50	Intensive chemotherapy and/or All-trans retinoic acid (ATRA) and arsenic trioxide Bone marrow transplant for relapsed APL	70% (trend improving with use of ATRA and arsenic)
Acute Lymphocytic Leukemia (ALL)	Cancer of the lymphoid cells in the bone marrow; cells grow uncontrollably (proliferate) and stop maturing (*blasts*—comprising 20% or more of the bone marrow).	6,000	16 (peaks in children and then again in older adults)	Intensive chemotherapy or Lower-dose chemotherapy or Watchful waiting Bone marrow transplant for high-risk ALL or for relapse	30% for adults (higher for good-risk features); 80–90% for children

Table 1.1 (continued)

Type of Leukemia	Description	Number of Yearly Diagnoses (US, estimated)	Median Age at Diagnosis (years)	Treatment	Five-Year Survival
Myelodysplastic Syndromes (MDS)	Cancer of the myeloid cells in the bone marrow; cells can be misshapen and grow uncontrollably (proliferate), and with advanced MDS stop maturing (blasts—comprising 19% or less of the bone marrow). Can transform to AML.	20,000	71	Lower-dose chemotherapy Bone marrow transplant for high-risk MDS or for relapse	30%

Table 1.1 (continued)

Type of Leukemia	Description	Number of Yearly Diagnoses (US, estimated)	Median Age at Diagnosis (years)	Treatment	Five-Year Survival
Chronic Myeloid Leukemia (CML)	Cancer of the myeloid cells in the bone marrow; in *chronic phase* CML, cells grow uncontrollably (proliferate) and with advanced CML stop maturing (blasts—comprising 19% or less of the bone marrow). Can transform to AML (called *blast crisis* CML).	9,000	65	Tyrosine kinase inhibitors (TKIs: imatinib, nilotinib, dasatinib, etc.)	70% (trend improving with use of TKIs)
Chronic Lymphocytic Leukemia (CLL)	Cancer of the lymphoid cells in the bone marrow; cells grow uncontrollably (proliferate) and with advanced CLL can transform to a large cell lymphoma or even ALL.	21,000	70	Lower-dose chemotherapy	85%

Myeloblasts, or just *blasts*, are primitive bone-marrow cells that eventually mature to become functional white blood cells. They are large, ugly, and menacing, particularly when they represent leukemia, and grow in sheets that seem to take over the other, normal bone marrow cells. Everyone has blasts in the bone marrow, but it is abnormal to have more than 5 percent of the bone-marrow contents consist of blasts. Once a person has 20 percent or more blasts, it indicates acute leukemia.

"What did Mr. Sweeney do for a living?" I asked next.

"He worked for a company that makes cardboard boxes." John answered quickly, obviously forewarned that I always ask about my patients' occupations. One colleague, a good friend of mine, wrote an essay about resilience in medicine, concluding that it boiled down to a "pathologic fascination with humanity."[6] I share that pathology—what buoys me is hearing about my patients' symptoms, their fears, their children and grandchildren, their hobbies, and yes, their occupations.

"A cardboard-box company?" I looked up from taking notes. "How do you make a cardboard box?" John looked at Becky, and then at me uncertainly, trying to discern whether I actually wanted him to respond. Was I asking seriously, or just teasing?

I continued with the questions. "What was his job in the factory? Did he enjoy his work?"

"I have no idea." This time, he answered a little more defensively. I couldn't blame him. He was post-call, had

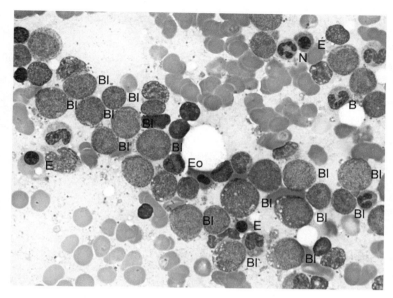

Figure 1.2

Large, menacing blasts in the bone marrow. This image shows a stained bone marrow aspirate smear from a patient with acute myeloid leukemia. Representative cells are identified (with the label placed to the right of each cell) as follows: Bl (blast), B (band neutrophil), N (segmented neutrophil), Eo (eosinophil), and E (erythroid). There are many blasts, cells with a large nucleus and scant cytoplasm (the sliver of space around the nucleus). Some normal, maturing white blood cells (B, N, Eo) and red blood cells (E) are present. Many light-colored mature red blood cells (erythrocytes) are visible in the background. *Source*: image courtesy of K. Theil, MD.

barely slept, and I was asking him if his patient *enjoyed* this line of work?

"Okay, let's rephrase the question. What was *your* worst job ever? And being an intern or resident doesn't count." The team laughed cautiously, and John looked at me, unsure again. Was he really supposed to answer?

Growing up in Rhode Island, I had my share of bad jobs. My first was at age 14 at a place called the Newport Creamery— basically, Friendly's with a Rhode Island twist. I worked on the grill and as a busboy, filling orders and clearing tables as quickly as possible. I cleaned bathrooms, followed OSHA rules, and learned to treat customers with respect. Not a terrible job, but I didn't have any basis for comparison.

The next year, I worked at a family-owned deli—that was a bad job. I even lied about my age so I could use the meat and cheese slicers, claiming I was 16. That was my first exposure to how dysfunctional staff can affect a workplace. The boss was moody, venting his anger by either insulting us or simply yelling. His wife, a mousy woman with a glass eye, did the accounting in the back room. The cook was addicted to cocaine and showed up sporadically. The boss's son, who was a party animal in college and barely graduated, worked behind the counter, despite having promised himself for years that he would never work in the old man's business. He had a tumultuous relationship with a woman who also worked behind the counter, and who would become unglued every time one of his former flames walked through the deli's front door—which occurred approximately every other day.

But the worst part of the job involved being sent to grab some extra jars of borscht from the basement. I would open the door leading downstairs, brace myself, flick on the light switch—and the floor would seem to move as the massive infestation of roaches scurried for cover. But again I learned, this time about working with people who did not get along and about completing tasks you don't particularly like, because it was my job. I also tried to see things from the boss's perspective—I mean, the boss wasn't exactly going to be like some Little Miss Sunshine, having worked in a disgusting deli his entire life.

Other jobs followed: many in food service but also as a truck driver, a maintenance man, and even in an ungodly hot warehouse at the peak of August. These jobs were not fun, but each gave me one more bit of knowledge about how a workplace functions, and how the things we take for granted are made. They also left me with a morbid curiosity about other people's jobs, how businesses operate, and about the process for making everyday objects.

"The witness is asked to answer the question. What was your worst job ever?" I persisted with John.

We went around, and each member of the team contributed. I have asked this question multiple times. Many residents have worked in labs before. Some have worked in offices or for their parents. One woman worked at a restaurant in New Jersey, and we shared our common knowledge about grill cleaning: You take a piece of window screen patch and place it flat on the hot grill, holding the patch with a towel. You then pour seltzer water on the surface, and press down as hard as you can while scrubbing. If you slip, you burn your knuckles. (We both have the scars to prove it.) Another woman, an intern, had worked alongside migrant workers in Idaho picking raspberries, and she described her arms at the end of the day, blood-streaked from the thorns on the bushes. That sounded like a bad job. These last two were probably the best residents I have ever supervised.

And the worst? They were the ones for whom internship was their first job. They were the ones who didn't understand why you have to check every lab, every vital sign, and every consultant's note—the ones who didn't understand that these tasks, as mundane as they are, actually have an impact on people's lives. And that it's their job to perform them.[7]

"Let's go in and chat with Mr. Sweeney," I suggested.

We walked into the hospital room. Mr. Sweeney was lying in bed, wearing a hospital gown patterned with the blue and green logo of our hospital. Diane von Furstenberg, who launched her brand in 1974 with a now-iconic wrap dress, had famously helped out with the design. He was slightly overweight, with a full head of hair, almost all salt with a dash of pepper. His legs were crossed causally, but his hand tapped the bed sheets nervously. A pole by his bed held a bag of saline, which dripped slowly through an IV in his arm. His wife sat in a chair by the window, in jeans and a scarlet and gray Ohio State sweatshirt. I introduced myself and asked each of the members of our team to introduce themselves. He asked me to call him David, and he introduced his wife, Betty.

"It's nice to meet you, and I'm sorry about the circumstances under which we're meeting," I said, as I sat in a chair by his bed. He nodded grimly in agreement. "Where are you from?"

"Ashtabula. Near Erie." Eastern part of the state, near the Pennsylvania border.

"Do you know why your doctor wanted you to be admitted to the hospital?"

"She wanted me to get treated for my condition," he answered. This time I nodded.

"And what condition is that?" I asked. I did not intend to be mean or to patronize him. But occasionally, and as bizarre as this sounds, our newly arrived patients aren't told that they have leukemia, but rather that they have a "blood" or "bone marrow" disorder. In one study we conducted, with almost 350 patients who had myelodysplastic syndromes, only 5 to 6 percent were told by their doctors that they had cancer or a condition similar to leukemia, whereas 80 percent were informed that they had a "blood condition"— despite the fact that their average survival was less than three years and most were treated with chemotherapy.[8]

David hesitated and glanced at his wife before saying the words. "Well, she says I have leukemia." His hand tapped the sheets a little quicker, as his wife pursed her lips.

"It's a scary word," I acknowledged. Without realizing it he had been holding his breath. As he exhaled, nodding in agreement, Betty started to cry. One of the interns rushed to get her a box of tissues. "Do you know what leukemia is?"

"It's a bone cancer," he said.

"That's right. Leukemia is a cancer of the bone marrow. Cancer involves the uncontrolled growth of cells. These cells acquire an abnormality that causes them to outgrow all of the normal cells around them. When this happens in the breast, a woman feels a lump. When it occurs in the lung, a person develops a mass that can be seen on an X-ray. The bone marrow is what I call a "high-rent district"—it can't expand like breast or lung tissue, so when cancer grows in it, that space fills up pretty quickly."

David was listening carefully as Betty put her tissue away, opened a small notebook, and prepared to take notes.

"Acute leukemia is unlike any other cancer in that two things actually happen: aside from the cells growing too fast, they also stop maturing. Imagine if the normal cells in your bone marrow started out as kindergarteners and keep maturing until they graduate high school, and then are pushed out into the blood stream to make a living as the white blood cells that fight infection, the red blood cells that deliver oxygen to the body's tissues, and the platelets that stop bleeding. As acute leukemia grows, the normal cells die out, leaving only kindergarteners, because the cancer cells stop maturing. Just as you wouldn't think that actual kindergarteners would function very well working in a factory or as carpenters, these cells can't build the white or red blood cells, or platelets, that the body needs. We call those kindergarteners 'blasts.'"

He nodded, recognizing the word from his hematologist's explanation of his bone marrow biopsy results.

"So how do you treat it?" Betty asked, her pen poised over her notepad.

This was a complicated question, perhaps more so than she had anticipated.

The standard, intensive chemotherapy treatment for AML is called "7+3." The "7" refers to the seven days of one chemotherapy drug, cytarabine, also called Ara-C, which was first isolated from Caribbean sponges and synthesized at the University of California, Berkeley, in 1959. It was approved by the FDA in 1969. The "3" refers to the three days of a second drug, daunorubicin, which derives from a microbe, *Streptomyces peucetius*, originally isolated from the soil surrounding a thirteenth-century castle (Castel del Monte) in Apulia, Italy, in the 1950s. The name *daunorubicin* is a combination of *Dauni*, a pre-Roman tribe that occupied the area where the compound was isolated; and *rubis*, which describes its red color. The FDA approved the drug in 1979.[9]

To understand how and why cytarabine and daunorubicin work, let's go back to what many of us learned in high school biology about mitosis, and about how cells divide. Mitosis starts in the cell's nucleus (its central portion) when DNA (the 23 pairs of chromosomes that are the blueprint for that particular cell's function) replicates. As mitosis continues, the cell makes a perfect copy of itself, including the newly replicated chromosomes. For the cell to copy its DNA, it must first relax the tightly coiled structures of the chromosomes, using an enzyme called topoisomerase. After the DNA is copied, it will return to its coiled state.

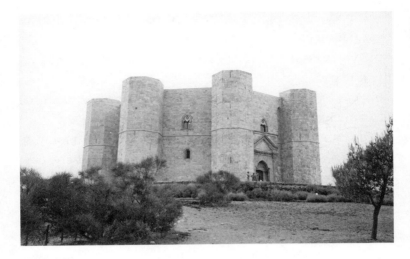

Figure 1.3
Castel del Monte, the castle around which the microbe *Streptomyces peuce-tius* was isolated.

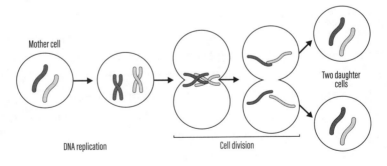

Figure 1.4
Mitosis, in which chromosomes replicate and the cell divides, making two perfect copies of itself. Topoisomerase helps relax the chromosomes so they can be copied (from 1st to 2nd step).

Cytarabine acts like a Trojan Horse with its resemblance to cytosine deoxyribose, the sugar used to build DNA. When cytarabine is administered to a person with leukemia, it is incorporated into the DNA instead of the cytosine, blocking the cell's ability to copy the DNA. (A cell that can't copy its DNA can't continue to grow and divide.) Cytarabine is given as a constant drip for 168 hours in a row. Daunorubicin, on the other hand, freezes the topoisomerase so the DNA cannot return to its coil, inhibiting the cell from copying itself. Daunorubicin is administered once daily as an intravenous "push" that lasts 10 minutes.

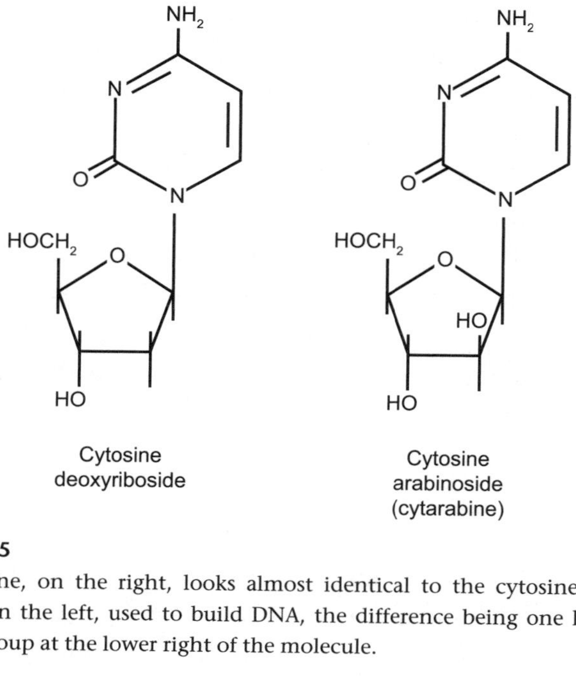

Cytosine
deoxyriboside

Cytosine
arabinoside
(cytarabine)

Figure 1.5
Cytarabine, on the right, looks almost identical to the cytosine deoxyribose, on the left, used to build DNA, the difference being one hydroxy (–OH) group at the lower right of the molecule.

Cancer cells, by definition, divide and copy themselves much more frequently than normal cells. That makes them exquisitely sensitive to the chemotherapy, as they are constantly trying to replicate their DNA. But other cells in the body that divide and copy themselves with some regularity—such as hair and skin cells, and the cells in the GI tract that replenish themselves every time we eat—also become susceptible to the chemo. This explains many of the chemotherapy's side effects: skin irritation and breakdown; hair loss; gastrointestinal events such as nausea, vomiting, diarrhea, and ulcers; and a precipitous drop in the blood counts (because the chemo also impairs the remaining normal bone marrow cells that continue to divide to make white and red blood cells and platelets). A person treated with 7+3 remains in the hospital for the seven days of chemotherapy, but also until the worst of the side effects have resolved—typically, for a total of a month or more.

The severity of the drug toxicities, and the body's ability to recover from them, limit the amount of chemotherapy we can give. For serious conditions like acute leukemia, we accept a lot more risk than we would for, say, a drug to treat high blood pressure, because the downside to not treating acute leukemia is so extreme: certain death, on average within two months.

I explained the treatment, hospital stay, and side effects to the Sweeneys. The members of my team, who had already heard several similar conversations taking place with other patients during the past week, were shuffling, leaning against the hospital wall, and in general growing restless. Routine for them, anything but routine for the Sweeneys.

So much of medicine has become mechanized, from the treatment pathways we recommend for a given condition, to our reliance on electronic medical records. When I bring my own children to see their pediatrician, I often see more of her back and shoulders, as she pecks away at the computer in her examination room to complete her office notes about them, than I do her face. She's under a lot of pressure, though, to complete those notes, or else she will have to take time away from her own children that night to finish them. One study found that primary care doctors spent almost 6 hours of an 11-hour workday populating information in the electronic medical record, 86 minutes of which was "pajama time"—after hours or at home.[10]

Facing someone with a new cancer diagnosis is different, though. Pathways make it easy to identify treatment options, and electronic medical records provide a simple way to order the right labs and prescribe the appropriate chemotherapy. But they can't determine a patient's goals, or read his body language.

"The chance that you could go into a remission, meaning we can't find the leukemia as hard as we look, is around 50 percent," I said. "But that isn't the same as cure. We only know for sure that you're cured of the leukemia when you come back to my outpatient clinic five years from now and it still hasn't returned."

Betty wrote down those numbers. "Then what's the chance you can cure it?" she asked.

I looked over to David, meeting him in the eyes. "Are these numbers you'd like to hear, or would you rather I talk in generalities?"

He shifted his legs, glanced over to his wife, and then looked back at me. "Let's hear it," he said.

"The chance that we can cure this leukemia in someone over the age of 60 is less than 10 percent. That number is low, but real. I have some folks, now in their 70s and 80s, who I can say are cured." I paused, letting the number sink in. David glanced down at his own hands as Betty wrote "<10%" in her notepad and then stopped writing, her eyes fixed on the pen still pressed to the paper.

"What's the chance I don't make it through this?" he asked.

"There are never guarantees," I acknowledged. "Because the chemotherapy will lower your immune system and your platelets, you can have infections or bleeding events that could be life threatening. The likelihood that you could die from the chemo is between 10 and 15 percent."

David mulled this over. "You're saying that I'm just as likely to be cured of the leukemia as to die from the chemotherapy. But if I don't take the chemo, then I'll definitely die from the leukemia." A statement, not a question. I nodded.

"It's a trade-off," I said. "You invest a month in the hospital, and risk dying, for a chance to live longer or even be cured. Or, you say to me, 'thanks but no thanks, doc' and leave the hospital, and we can give you lower-dose chemo as an outpatient or support you with blood and platelet transfusions, as you need them."

"And that low-dose chemotherapy, can it cure him?" Betty asked. I shook my head.

"No. It has about a 15 to 20 percent chance of getting you into a remission. And the people who enter a remission— either with low-dose or intense chemotherapy—live longer than those who don't go into a remission. But it isn't curative." She wrote down the numbers.

"This is a hard decision," David commented. I wished I could have guided him better.

Unfortunately, the last time a clinical trial compared giving older adults intensive chemotherapy versus low-dose therapy or supportive care was in the late 1980s. Other studies—deemed "retrospective"—have looked back at how patients fared when treated with intensive or low-dose chemotherapy, but not as part of a formal trial. Those studies had mixed results, with some showing an advantage to intensive chemotherapy, and some showing no difference for intensive chemotherapy versus low-dose chemo or supportive care.[11] The problem with those retrospective studies is what's called a selection bias—that healthier patients were more likely to have been treated with intensive chemotherapy than unhealthy patients, and thus to have had a better outcome. The better outcome may have been because they were healthier to start with, and not because of any impact of the chemotherapy.

"Why don't you take some time today to think it over?" I suggested. "There's no wrong answer of what to choose— only what feels right to you, what your gut tells you."

The Sweeneys nodded their agreement and thanked us for coming in. It always amazes me, how in this life-altering moment, my patients retain such kindness to be thankful when I have given them such rotten news. I rose from my chair to leave, but hesitated.

"I'm sorry, just one more question," I said, as I motioned toward the post-call resident. "John tells me that you worked for a cardboard-box manufacturer."

"That's right, in a factory in Erie," David replied.

"How many years?"

"Oh, goin' on about 25 or 30. You don't see many people sticking that long with a company anymore," he reflected.

I agreed. "How exactly do you make a cardboard box?"

He shifted to sit up higher in his bed. "We make the cardboard itself out of wood pulp. Then the sides of the box are glued together using a starch," he explained.

"Is that factory operational seven days a week?"

"Oh no," he laughed. "There's not that much of an urgent need for cardboard boxes! We were closed on the weekends. The problem was, that starch would go bad if it wasn't used, so over the weekends, we added a preservative to the starch so it was still good on Monday."

"Any idea what that preservative was made of?" I asked.

"Oh yeah," David said. "It was made of formaldehyde."

Formaldehyde. A known carcinogen linked to leukemia.[12]

2
A Bleak Start to Life

> *. . . Born in a time*
> *of darkness, you will learn the trick of making.*
> *You shall make your consolation all your life.*
> —Amanda Jernigan, "Lullaby," 2005

"Our next patient is a transfer from Obstetrics." The junior resident John said, as I left Mr. Sweeney's room. Our eyes locked for a second as we shared our mutual worry.

"What trimester is she?" I asked.

"Second."

I nodded and exhaled. "Well, at least she has that going for her."

Cancer is always a serious diagnosis. Leukemia is a serious cancer diagnosis. Leukemia in a woman who is pregnant takes on a whole other level of danger, for a couple of reasons.

First, leukemia cripples the immune system's ability to fight infections, and the chemotherapy we give to treat the leukemia just makes the immune system all that much worse. Pregnancy can also impair the immune system, albeit mildly. But add that to an immune system already on the ropes from leukemia, and the risk of acquiring a life-threatening infection becomes much higher.

Second, the chemotherapy I described to the Sweeneys could cause severe birth defects in an unborn child, or worse. The likelihood that a woman would be able to keep her baby if this had occurred during the first trimester was nil. The chemotherapy, which works by killing growing cancer cells (remember the Trojan Horse cytarabine), crosses the placenta and instead kills the rapidly dividing cells in a fetus that is trying to grow limbs and organs. During the second trimester, when the cells aren't dividing quite as much, there would be a chance for the baby to survive, though risks of birth defects and fetal death were still quite high.

I carry around my own baggage regarding pregnant women with leukemia. My very first month of being a staff physician, right after my fellowship training, I cared for a pregnant woman who was also in her second trimester. She had acute lymphoblastic leukemia, which can affect the bone marrow cells like acute myeloid leukemia but can also, rarely, grow as solid tumors almost anywhere in the body. In fact, her leukemia was diagnosed when she was undergoing a routine ultrasound of her baby and the radiology technician noticed a mass on one of her kidneys, nearby the uterus. It was biopsied, leukemia was diagnosed, and she was admitted to my service.

We started chemotherapy and asked the Obstetrics team to round on her every day and to perform ultrasounds on the unborn child. Boy, did she look great, teasing us and telling jokes during rounds every morning. The baby was doing wonderfully, too. She taped ultrasound photos of her baby on her hospital wall, which buoyed all of our spirits, and reminded us of what was at stake here.

But then, one week into her treatment, she spiked a fever. That morning when I went in to see her, she looked worried for the first time since I had met her.

"Something's wrong. Something's really wrong," she told me. Even at that early stage of my career, I had enough sense to trust my patients when they told me there was a significant change in their well-being. I looked down at her legs, which stuck out from under the bed sheets, and saw livedo—a medical term for when a body part looks mottled, as if it has lost some essence of life. It is frequently associated with sepsis—an infection that has entered the blood stream and is starting to wreak havoc with the body.

"We'll take care of you," I told her, trying to reassure her as much as myself. But I was worried too.

We gave her antibiotics immediately, but within 2 hours she had to be transferred to the intensive care unit because her blood pressure dropped. Within 8 hours, she had been placed on a ventilator. At 12 hours after the fever started, the baby had died. By hour 18, she too had died.

"Ms. Badway is a 36-year-old woman who is G6 P3"— shorthand for "gravida 6 para 3," meaning she has been pregnant six times and has delivered three children. "She went to see her OB at week 20 of her pregnancy when a routine CBC showed a white blood cell count of 330,000, a hemoglobin of 10.3, and a platelet count of 470,000."

"Wait," I interrupted John. "Did you say her platelet count was 470,000?" He nodded. "That's high. The hemoglobin's a bit high too. It's pretty unusual for someone with acute leukemia to have preserved platelet counts." Joan's numbers—with a hemoglobin near 7 and a platelet count south of 20—were far more typical. I started to feel a glimmer of hope. Maybe Ms. Badway didn't have acute leukemia after all.

John, along with the rest of the team, stared at me, not sure where I was going with this. Rachel, a hematology/oncology fellow who was in her second year of training *after* her three years of internal medicine residency, emerged from Ms. Badway's room. I assumed she had just performed a bone marrow biopsy, as she stripped off a blue paper surgical gown, crumbled it into a ball, and threw it in the trash. She put her white coat back on and joined us.

Bone marrow biopsies have been used to evaluate disease causes for more than a century. The contemporary biopsy needle was invented by the Iranian hematologist Khosrow Jamshidi in 1971. This is the procedure we follow: We stick the needle into the flat part of the pelvis, in the back and just below the spine, and remove some of the marrow so a pathologist can analyze it. We choose the pelvis because it contains some of the most fertile bone marrow "soil" in the body. The biopsy needle is almost comically long, as it needs to reach the bone that is sometimes buried deeply beneath the skin. A few years ago, I probably forfeited any parent-of-the-year aspirations I had by bringing one as a visual aid to my son's elementary school when I taught his classmates how blood was made. Looking at the needle, which evokes a prop for a movie about a mad scientist, they unsurprisingly recoiled at its size. Two of his horrified classmates even asked to leave the room.

The needle has recently been replaced by a drill that was shown in one study to work just as well and to cause less discomfort.[1] Though anecdotally some patients have told me they feel less pain with the drill, others say it gives them even more anxiety, as they associate it with sounds they normally hear when thrust into an uncomfortable position in a dentist's chair.

"How'd the biopsy go?" I asked Rachel.

"It was a little tricky. She couldn't lay on her stomach because of the pregnancy, but we were able to prop her up to lay on her side with pillows, and I think we got a good sample."

I followed up by asking, "Did you learn anything else about Ms. Badway while you were in there?"

"Well, I know she doesn't work for a cardboard box company." We all laughed.

"John, can you read off the blood counts again to Rachel?" He repeated them. "What do you think Rachel?" I asked.

She considered the lab results for a second and asked him, "What was the patient's differential?" The differential is a description of the subtypes of white blood cells that appear in the blood stream. Normally, it consists mainly of neutrophils (around 60 percent of the white blood cells), which fight bacterial infections; lymphocytes (around 30 percent), which attack viruses; and maybe a few eosinophils, which become elevated when we have allergies, or monocytes, which attack atypical infections like tuberculosis. With acute leukemia, the differential shifts markedly: we might see 1 percent neutrophils, 10 percent lymphocytes, and 89 percent of those blasts that started their lives in the bone marrow.

John started reading a string of percentages from the computer on his WOW: "neutrophils (50), lymphocytes (15), eosinophils (10), monocytes (6), basophils (8), promyelocytes (7), metamyelocytes (2), and blasts (2)." He looked up, first at Rachel and then at me, waiting for us to interpret what he had just said.

"Are you worried about those blasts, Rachel? Should we start her on daunorubicin and cytarabine, like Mr. Sweeney?" I asked, knowing she was too smart to be tricked by the leading question.

She crinkled her nose. "This sounds much more like a myeloproliferative disorder. Could it be CML?"

I nodded. "I think that's exactly what it is, which is great news for her."

Myeloproliferative disorders, as the name implies, occur when the myeloid cells in the bone marrow grow (proliferate) rapidly. Unlike acute leukemia, in which the immature blasts—the kindergarteners—grow too fast because they stop maturing, with myeloproliferative disorders, more advanced stages in bone marrow cell development (promyelocytes, metamyelocytes, basophils, neutrophils) grow too fast—call them the high schoolers. That was the explanation for Ms. Badway's unusual differential.

Here's the really odd thing about myeloproliferative disorders: for some reason we don't quite understand, the rapidly growing cells also release chemicals in the bone marrow. Those chemicals can eventually lead to a type of scar tissue called *fibrosis* accumulating within that high-rent, precious space. The remaining normal bone marrow cells recognize that their home is rapidly becoming inhospitable. So they decide to get the heck out of Dodge and find somewhere else in the body to reside.

When we were all at the developing fetus stage, none of us actually had a functional bone marrow. Instead, those bone marrow cells created red blood cells, white blood cells, and platelets from what's called our reticuloendothelial system— the liver, spleen, and lymph nodes. Remarkably, in people with myeloproliferative disorders, the bone marrow cells somehow remember where they were born, even decades later, and return to those organs as safe havens when the disease worsens. Consequently, people with these disorders often have enlarged spleens, livers, or lymph nodes. Blood passing through these organs picks up some of the young progeny of the bone marrow cells, and thus the reason for the unusual white blood cells in Ms. Badway's differential.

"Let's go in and chat with Ms. Badway," I said to the team after they told me a little more about her medical history.

"She asked if she could just talk to you and me," Rachel interjected. "There was a lot of traffic in and out of her room overnight." I could just imagine it: the registered nurse who would have admitted her, the licensed practicing nurse who would have taken her vital signs every couple of hours, the on-call resident, and then, crossing the 7 a.m. shift change, a whole new crew of nurses and residents—then Rachel, and now me.

We walked into her room, Rachel leading me, as she had already met our new patient. Ms. Badway was lying in bed, sleeping on her side. No surprise, given what must have been a busy night and the pain medications we administer prior to a bone marrow biopsy. She was wearing black sweatpants and a matching, zippered sweatshirt. Her designer hospital gown and an extra pair of bed sheets lay carefully folded on the windowsill.

A lot of my patients won't wear a gown for a number of days into their hospital admission—some because their street clothes are simply more comfortable; some because they still can't believe they have a leukemia diagnosis and aren't ready to dress as if they are ill; and still others to remind themselves what life outside the hospital feels like. Sun streamed through the windows in a rare break from the slate gray skies that blanket Cleveland every fall and only rarely lift before late April. The skyline, two miles away, looked magnificent.

Rachel gently rubbed Ms. Badway's leg and called her name. She sat up in bed and Rachel introduced me.

"Hi," I said, sitting at the edge of her bed.

"Hey," she answered, rubbing the sleep from her eyes. "So, you're the guy who's going to make all of this better?"

"Well, we're sure going to try," I answered. "Did Rachel talk to you about what's going on?" She nodded. "How do you feel?"

"That's the crazy thing!" she almost shouted. "I feel fine. I mean, don't get me wrong. I'm pregnant and all, and after barfing for three months now I get to be just exhausted and fat. My clothes not fitting, that sucks. And it doesn't help that I've got three kids at home who are pains in my ass. My husband Joe is with them now. Especially my daughter, who is in high school where the only thing she seems to learn is how to push my buttons." She paused, as if contrasting the routine of her life—and what she might have characterized as "frustrating" 24 hours earlier—to where she was right now. "But leukemia? No way."

She looked at me, waiting for me to agree with her, that it was impossible that she could have leukemia.

"We're going to find out one way or the other what is making your blood counts so abnormal. That's why Rachel attacked you with a big needle just now," I said.

"This is insane. This can't be happening." She shook her head again. "You don't understand, my life is finally settling out. Before this . . ." She shook her head again. "You wouldn't want any part of me."

"What do you mean?"

She looked me in the eyes, defiantly this time. "I was bad news. I first met Joe in high school, but I was too much of a wild child even for him!" She laughed. "Back then it was just a lot of drinking. And pot. Landed me in the emergency room a couple of times to get my stomach pumped, when I was at Tri-C." The Cuyahoga Community College. "But I only lasted there a couple of years. School wasn't really for me. So a girlfriend of mine got me a job dancing."

"Dancing?" I asked. "What kind?"

A smile crept over her face, and she looked at me with pity for all those years I had kept my nose stuffed in medical textbooks. "Of the pole variety. At the Crazy Horse, downtown. Those were some rough times. The drinking got pretty bad, too, until one time I was at this party and fell out a window and landed on my back. I fell two stories. Broke my pelvis." John had alluded to some past trauma she had sustained. "That scared me straight. I quit the Crazy Horse. Finished school at Tri-C. And then Joe came back into my life." She smiled again, but fleetingly. "And now this."

I nodded, holding her gaze but fighting the urge to say anything. It's such a normal, even empathic human tendency, to want to fill these spaces in conversation with reassuring words, to somehow take this weight—of her past life, her present life as a busy mom, her pregnancy, and now her leukemia—off her shoulders. Studies in which doctor-patient interactions are observed have found that, on average, we interrupt patients after they have been talking for only 11 seconds when they are trying to tell us their stories, and perhaps clue us in on what led to the illnesses that have altered their lives.[2] So we sat together, in silence, as she processed where she was in the world.

Eventually she sighed. "So tell me what's the next step. I gotta get this fixed so I can get back home and take care of my rotten kids." She started to cry. Rachel grabbed the tissue box and handed it to her. The tissues were part of our daily routine.

"We're worried that you have leukemia," I answered. "We don't mess around even when we just suspect it, and that's why you came straight to our floor. But there are a couple of flavors of leukemia: the acute kind, which we do consider a medical emergency, and which would require immediate chemotherapy and a stay here of four to six weeks . . ."

Her eyes widened at the thought, and if she was like any other parent of school-age children I had treated, she was probably trying to figure out how their lives would stay on track if she were incapacitated in the hospital. I'm sure it was no easy feat just for her to be admitted and for her husband to stay home from work for the day.

". . . and the chronic kind, which can be treated as an outpatient, actually with chemotherapy pills. We have some early results from your blood counts, and they seem more typical of the latter, the chronic form of leukemia. *Chronic myeloid leukemia, CML.*" I said the words deliberately because other patients have told me how meaningful it was, that initial time when I gave their leukemia a name. "I'm keeping my fingers crossed that we're right." I smiled at her.

"Yeah, me too," she said, thinking over what I had just told her. "Any idea what caused it? Was it the drugs and the booze?"

Scores of my patients have posed a similar question to me, wondering about a cause.[3] I suppose it reflects an innate need to revisit whether all the small decisions we make, about the foods we eat, the habits in which we indulge, and the steps we should have taken to mitigate harm, could have avoided an untoward outcome.

But truthfully, except in very obvious cases, it is difficult to determine if a specific environmental exposure triggered a person's cancer. Most cancers arise spontaneously, as if thumbing their nose at our primal need to establish a cause.

But I still try, as the residents learned with Mr. Sweeney. And sometimes, I even convince myself that, like some sorcerer of truth, I have uncovered THE EVENT that caused the cancer.

One patient with myelodysplastic syndrome told me she used to live in Nevada. I asked her whether she had been exposed to any chemicals or radiation.

"Well," she said, laughing to herself, as if marveling at the foolishness of what she was about to tell me. "Our family lived there when I was a girl, in the 1950s. Every so often, someone in the town posted flyers on the telephone poles inviting us to gather outside and watch the mushroom cloud that would follow the nuclear bomb testing nearby. That was big entertainment!" She laughed. "So we'd all wait for the big explosion, and then as the cloud formed, the hot winds from it would blow through the town, and almost knock us over."

I imagined the radioactive noxious breeze, encircling her impressionable bone marrow stem cells when she was just a girl.

Another time, a man in his 70s with acute leukemia told me he'd served in the navy. I asked him if he'd seen any action.

"I was on a ship during the Cuban Missile Crisis," he said, shaking his head. "It was hotter 'n hell down there. And humid."

I laughed. "Wow! That's incredible. How'd you stay cool?"

"I didn't!" This time *he* laughed. "Except at night. Instead of lying in our bunks, a couple of guys and I would lug a mattress down to the hull and lay it on the ground, in between some metal cases that were cool at night. We kept the nuclear weapons in those cases."

Nuclear arsenal only a foot or two from his bone marrow? Perhaps this exposure, half a century earlier, was the culprit.

I've had patients who worked in shoe stores and used fluoroscopy (X-ray) imaging to visualize the bones in a customer's foot. This popular gimmick, used from the 1930s to the 1950s or so, was said to help determine the right shoe size—but no one, neither shopkeeper nor customer, wore a lead vest for protection. Other patients employed by a well-known tire manufacturer south of Cleveland described to me how they would soak their hands, for hours at a time, in a vat of benzene, similar to the formaldehyde Mr. Sweeney mentioned.

Doctors themselves recommended similar exposures before they recognized the downstream consequences of their treatment. My uncle had the acne on his back treated with radiation in the late 1940s, when he was a teenager. He died of leukemia in his 70s.

It is true that environmental factors can cause CML, but recreational drugs and alcohol have not been linked to this cancer (though alcohol does increase the chance of developing head and neck cancers). Most cases arise spontaneously, the exception being in people exposed to the atomic bombs the United States dropped on Japan in 1945.

Although it seems intuitive now that people exposed to the atomic bombs would be at higher risk for cancer, that was not the case in real time. It took the death of a 12-year-old girl named Sadako Sasaki to bring attention to the hibakusha, the survivors of the bombings at Hiroshima and Nagasaki. Before she died of leukemia in 1955, she folded 1,000 origami cranes as a response to a legend that doing so would grant her a wish. The cranes have subsequently become a symbol of the victims of nuclear warfare.

The Atomic Bomb Disease Institute, subsequently established in 1962 in Nagasaki, Japan, conducts basic research in radiation medicine and the late effects of radiation on the human body. Ten years later, the Medical Data Center for the Atomic Bomb was established with the purpose of data collection and arrangement and preservation of materials from atomic bomb victims to better understand the effects of the disaster. These materials include information on precisely where each person was located in relation to the bomb's epicenter, which allows scientists to calculate how much radiation that person was exposed to.[4]

Some early studies (done in the 1980s) saw a spike in survivors having CML in the years immediately following 1945, but those numbers leveled off to almost normal thereafter.[5] In another study, scientists from the Atomic Bomb Disease Institute reported the incidence of myelodysplastic syndrome, diagnosed between 1985 and 2004, 40 to 60 years after the atomic bomb explosion. As you might expect, people who were younger and received higher doses of radiation because they were closer to the explosion were at highest risk of developing the cancer. The average age at the time of exposure to radiation was 9 years, and at the time of the myelodysplastic syndrome diagnosis the average age was 71 years. In other words, the radiation set in motion the first step of developing a cancer that wouldn't become manifest until decades later.[6]

Another example of an environmental cause is therapeutic radiation exposure. I have also cared for patients who developed CML decades after being treated with radiation therapy for Hodgkin lymphoma.

Hodgkin's was one of the first successfully treated cancers ever. People like Henry Kaplan, considered one of the pioneers in radiation therapy for cancer during his years at Stanford University, were considered heroes in the 1950s and 1960s for doing what was thought impossible: helping people with a cancer diagnosis to survive for years, and even to be cured. The timing and location of his work were not an accident: he co-opted the linear accelerators required to deliver radiation with the help of the Stanford physicists who had developed and used the technology to create the atomic bombs.

This initial euphoria around the success of radiation therapy was tempered when, years later, patients returned to Dr. Kaplan's clinic with new cancers: cancers of the skin and soft tissues (sarcomas) in the areas overlying the cancer-containing lymph nodes treated with the radiation; breast cancers, if those treated lymph nodes were deep in the chest, behind the breasts; and leukemias, when the radiation struck the bone marrow. Henry Kaplan suffered a deep depression afterward, when he realized that his treatment had caused significant enough genetic damage in normal cells in the body to make them cancerous. And not just cancerous—deadly. Cancers that arise as a result of treating other cancers, with radiation therapy or chemotherapy (which also can damage normal cells), are often the hardest to cure.[7]

I asked one patient who had been diagnosed with CML decades after her treatment for Hodgkin's lymphoma if she had any regrets, facing leukemia long after she was cured of her lymphoma.

She shook her head immediately and smiled at me. "No way. None. I have two beautiful children now, who I never would have had otherwise, and a loving husband. I've had an incredible life." She paused then, as if revisiting all that had transpired since her lymphoma diagnosis. "And I'm the only one still alive, out of all those people in the waiting room from when I was treated. The only one."

I reassured Ms. Badway that neither booze and drugs, nor any of her past activities, had caused the leukemia.

She exhaled, relieved, not so much for herself, I guessed, but because she didn't want to haunt her family with the thought that her previous behavior had so drastically affected her health.

"Okay, next question. What about the baby, can he get it?"

I remembered John telling me that she was having a boy.

"The short answer is no." I hesitated before answering, and she picked up on that.

"Gimme the long answer," she said. I liked her. No non-sense. Street smart. And she had lived a life, despite only being in her mid-thirties.

There are three ways in which a child can theoretically "get" a parent's leukemia: the child and the parent can all be exposed to the same radiation or chemical (as might happen to a family living near ground zero in Hiroshima in 1945) and contract the same cancer, which would be very unusual; the child can inherit it; or it can be passed from parent to child.

Leukemia can run in families as a heritable genetic predisposition, but it is exceptionally rare. In my decade-and-a-half of practice, I might have referred a patient approximately once every year or two for genetic counseling to determine if that patient had a chance of passing cancer on to children and grandchildren.

I did take care of one patient, a man in his mid-60s, who told me his identical twin brother also had leukemia, and that his father had died of leukemia. His brother came to see me too, and both donated blood samples for our research team to analyze. We discovered that they shared the same genetic abnormality and that they had both inherited it. (We can distinguish genetic abnormalities someone is born with and thus can pass on to children, called *germline* mutations, from those that are acquired randomly or from environmental exposures, called *somatic* mutations.) Both had leukemia that improved to a specific drug, too, and when we went back to our database of genetic abnormalities in people with leukemia and identified those who had the same genetic abnormality as these brothers, all improved if they had been treated with the same drug. It was remarkable.[8]

Classically, cancers that run in families tend to strike when people are young. Some cancers require that multiple genetic errors must occur before the cancer becomes manifest, though. And we are learning, as my twin-brother patients illustrate, that for those multiple genetic error cancers, like myelodysplastic syndromes or acute leukemias, they may run in families even when the cancer strikes at advanced ages. The germline mutation is just the first genetic step of many.

Cancers can be passed from parent to child, or one person to another, but again this is exceptionally rare. There are a few case reports in the medical literature of a person receiving a solid organ transplant from a donor—say, a heart, kidney, or even liver—and developing cancer in the months following the transplant.[9] That cancer can be linked back genetically to the donor. And although a detailed medical history is obtained from the donor's medical record and family at the time of organ donation, and the surgeons removing an organ from a donor look for any signs of obvious cancer, that donor was likely carrying a cancer that was still in its microscopic stages, only blossoming when placed in another person's body.

Only a couple of case reports, ever, have documented leukemia passing from a pregnant woman to her unborn child.[10] The placenta serves as a barrier between mother and child, protecting the fetus from much of what occurs in the mother's body, and vice versa. But it isn't a perfect system. As any pregnant woman who eats a sugary dessert and reports her baby "rockin' and rollin'" afterward can tell you, the baby gets the sugar load too. Blood cells can pass back and forth between mother and infant across the placenta, which means so could leukemia. Despite that, for the thousands of women who have had cancer while pregnant, to only have a couple of case reports of *vertical transmission* of cancer, the placental barrier must work pretty well.

I explained all of this to Ms. Badway, and asked her if she had any other questions.

"When will we know for sure what I have?" she wondered. She was rubbing her belly gently, as if reassuring her son that he would be okay.

"We should hear back from the pathologists this afternoon. As soon as we know, you'll know."

She thanked us and we left her room to finish rounds.

"Let's take a field trip," I suggested to our team after we had seen our final patient. "I wonder if those bone marrows are ready for our viewing pleasure."

We took the stairs down to the second floor, and then followed one connecting hallway to another, over Carnegie Avenue, through the entrance to the old Packard automobile dealership building, which houses our pathology department. Down some more stairs to the basement, through a locked door that my ID badge sometimes opens, and sometimes doesn't, and down another hall to the farthest room. This is where the multiheaded microscopes live—they make it possible for a group to examine the same slide at the same time—and where the bone marrow biopsy specimens are evaluated.

Karl, one of my favorite pathologists, was sitting by one of the scopes. He has a few years on me, both at our hospital and in life, and he remains one of the most thoughtful and gentle people I know. Outside of work, he collects player pianos, of all things. He is a renowned morphologist, meaning he can look at the shape of cells in the bone marrow—along with their numbers, where they are located, and what they look like in relation to each other—and almost invariably come up with the right diagnosis before additional, specialized test results returned.

"I bet I know why you're here," he said, smiling at me. "Business always seems to be good when you're on-service."

"That's good news / bad news," I answered, grimly. "I'd love to have treatments that put us both out of business, Karl."

He nodded in agreement. "So, would you like to review the bone marrow slides from Mr. Sweeney first, or the new gal with CML?"

"Does she have CML for sure?" I asked.

"Well, it sure looks like it. Of course, we'll have to wait for the tests to come back to see if she's *BCR-ABL* positive." He pulled out a thick cardboard panel from a stack of them on his desk and opened the front flaps. It looked like one of those old cardboard displays that held coins tucked into individual flaps, or like an Advent calendar board. But instead of coins, it held slides, each with a smudge of pink at the center. Karl picked one out and placed it under his microscope. We all gathered around one of the other two microscope heads. Karl walked us through the different cell types quickly, moving the slide around expertly, and efficiently increasing the magnification of the lens on the scope to make the cells bigger and bigger.

"Ninety-five percent cellular, here you see some myelocytes, metamyelocytes, eosinophils, band neutrophils. Here's even a blast," he said, identifying the large, pink and purple-colored blobs that would become mature white blood cells and red blood cells. "I'm counting only 1 percent blasts. These cells are pretty mature. There's a lot of them," he commented. "Classic bone marrow aspirate for CML."

We lifted our heads from the microscope as Karl grabbed another cardboard folder.

"Now this young man," he said, referring to Mr. Sweeney, "he has a lot of these." He stopped, as a scrum of large,

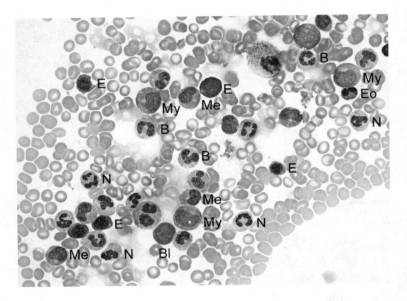

Figure 2.1
This image shows a stained bone marrow aspirate smear from a patient with chronic myeloid leukemia. Representative cells are identified (with the label placed to the right of each cell, with the exception Bl, labeled below cell) as follows: Bl (blast), My (myelocyte), Me (metamyelocyte), B (band neutrophil), N (segmented neutrophil), Eo (eosinophil). There are many more myeloid (Bl, My, Me, B, N, Eo) than erythroid (E) cells. Many mature, light-colored red blood cells (erythrocytes) are visible in the background. *Source*: image courtesy of K. Theil, MD.

menacing, irregularly shaped cells crowded almost half of the microscope's viewing field. Blasts.

"What percentage are you getting?" I asked, knowing the answer but hoping Karl would give me a different number.

"Between 40 and 45 percent," he answered. "I did a 500-cell count." Meaning, he went above and beyond what was standard, a 200-cell count, in which he literally counts the different cell types and adds up the percentages for 200 or 500 cells. "I'm sorry," he said. That's one thing I love about Karl. He knew that behind these slide there were people whose lives had just changed drastically for the worse.

"Thanks for taking some time out with us," I responded.

"I heard through the grapevine another is on the way?" He was alluding to Joan Walker. I nodded. "We'll be waiting for her."

As we headed back to the floor I said to the team, "Let's go tell Ms. Badway the good news." Well, relatively good news. I shook my head, reflecting on my own callousness. She still had leukemia, just not acute leukemia.

CML is defined by a specific genetic abnormality—what Karl referred to as the *BCR-ABL* translocation, in which chromosomes 9 and 22 switch "legs" with each other. (The first part of the abbreviation stands for "breakpoint cluster region," and the second part is shorthand for the Abelson oncogene, initially discovered by Herbert Abelson in 1970.)

Our DNA is housed in 23 pairs of chromosomes numbered from 1 to 22 (the 23rd being a pair of sex chromosomes designated as either XX for women or XY for men). During mitosis, as our genes make copies of themselves, the duplicate pairs of chromosomes all gather in the middle of the cell, as if they are line dancing. The cell then pinches itself in the middle and separates into two cells, with half of the chromosomes going one direction into one new cell, and half the other direction into the second cell.

But cells don't always make perfect copies of themselves, or of their chromosomes and DNA. Occasionally, chromosomes next to each other will trade genetic material. And when that trade gives a cell a growth advantage compared to other cells around it, cancer may result.

The field of human genetics began with the discovery of the 23 chromosome pairs in 1956. In 1960 a team of researchers, Peter Nowell and David Hungerford, obtained bone marrow samples from patients admitted to Philadelphia General Hospital in the late 1950s.

They noticed that seven patients with CML had cells with a normal number of chromosomes, but that one was shortened—chromosome 22, which became known as the *Philadelphia chromosome*.[11] This was the first time a genetic abnormality was consistently linked to cancer. Actually, what they didn't notice was that another chromosome, 9, had extra genetic material that came from chromosome 22.

So for more than 10 years, CML was thought to come from a *loss* of genetic material in the Philadelphia chromosome. It wasn't until 1972 that Janet Rowley, at the University of Chicago, showed that the Philadelphia chromosome resulted from a translocation—a switching of genetic material—between chromosome 9 and chromosome.[12]

It took almost another 20 years for researchers, led by George Daly and the Nobel laureate David Baltimore, to show that introducing this translocation to genetic material in mice caused CML to occur in the rodents.

Why was it important to give mice leukemia? Two reasons. First, it proved that the genetic abnormality alone

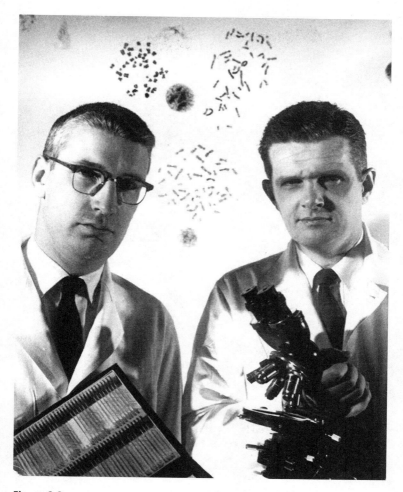

Figure 2.2
Peter Nowell and David Hungerford, who discovered the Philadelphia chromosome, pictured in 1961.

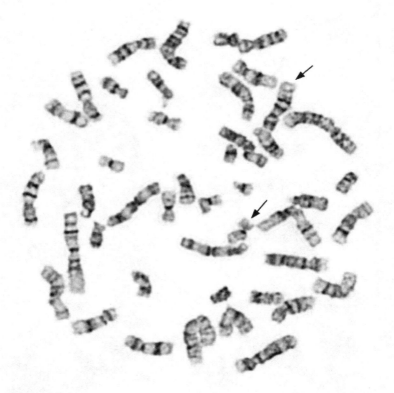

Figure 2.3
This image, from a male patient with CML, shows stained ("banded") chromosomes from a single cell frozen in mitosis. Arrows point to the abnormal chromosomes 9 and 22. These two chromosomes have exchanged material resulting in a longer chromosome 9, and a shorter chromosome 22, compared to their normal partners; the shortened chromosome 22 is known as the Philadelphia chromosome. *Source*: image courtesy of K. Theil, MD.

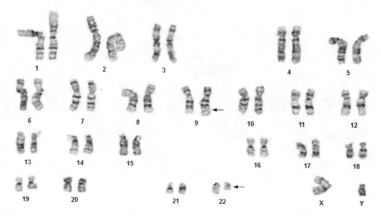

Figure 2.4

This image, known as a karyogram, was prepared from the same cell and shows chromosomes matched up as pairs arranged in order according to a conventional standard. There are 22 pairs of autosomes (chromosomes 1–22) and one pair of sex chromosomes (XY in this male patient). In the pair of chromosomes marked 9, the chromosome on the right is slightly longer indicating excess chromosome material from chromosome 22. In the pair of chromosomes marked 22, the chromosome on the right is slightly shorter, indicating a loss of chromosome material, given to chromosome 9. An arrow indicates the site on the abnormal chromosomes 9 and 22 where each has swapped (translocated) material with the other. *Source*: image courtesy of K. Theil, MD.

was enough to cause the disease. Unlike acute leukemia or myelodysplastic syndromes, which required multiple genetic abnormalities to occur before the cancer blossomed, CML was a "one-hit wonder." And second, now investigators had a small mammal with the same disease, in which they could test drugs to see if they could beat back the leukemia.

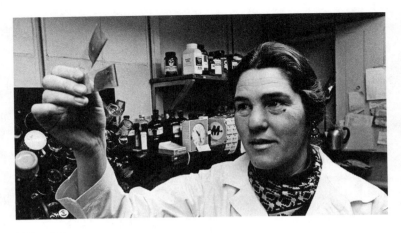

Figure 2.5
Janet Rowley, who first showed that the Philadelphia chromosome resulted from a translocation of chromosomes 9 and 22, working in her laboratory in the 1980s. *Source*: photo courtesy of University of Chicago, the *Chicago Maroon*.

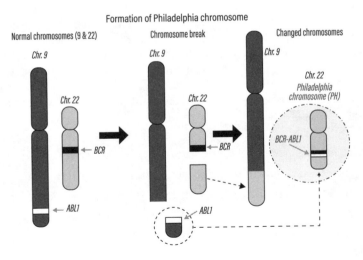

Figure 2.6
The translocation of chromosomes 9 and 22, creating the Philadelphia chromosome *BCR-ABL*.

Rachel entered Ms. Badway's room again, where she sat in a chair, sending a text message. The window now framed clouds, which had moved in to displace the sun.

"Just finishing this up," she said to us, distractedly. "Joe got the older kids off to school but forgot to pack their lunches. Hopefully they're at least wearing clothes." Leukemia or not, she had a household to run. She shut off her phone and looked up at us. I sat at the edge of her bed. "Okay, waddaya got for me?"

"We just took a look at the samples from your bone marrow, with our pathologist. It looks like you have chronic myeloid leukemia, not the acute leukemia we were worried about. This is good news," I told her, despite myself.

"The chronic leukemia." She repeated, processing what I told her. I nodded. "The one where I can go home?"

"That's right. We can actually send you home later this afternoon." I smiled. She didn't smile back, still thinking through the implications of this new information.

"Does that mean this isn't serious?"

I paused before answering. "It's still a serious diagnosis, and to be honest, we aren't 100 percent sure of the diagnosis yet. I'd put us at about 90 percent. We're waiting for another test to come back to be absolutely confident, and we'll get those results in a couple of days. But I'm comfortable enough at 90 percent to recommend you start taking the chemotherapy pills that work for this leukemia."

"And what exactly is the treatment for the chronic leukemia?" she asked.

Twenty years earlier, if I had faced the same question by a patient in her mid-30s, I would have answered without hesitation "a bone marrow transplant." With this procedure, a patient with CML receives a high dose of chemotherapy to essentially obliterate her bone marrow, and then receives another person's healthy bone marrow, which then takes up residence in her now-empty marrow space to produce new blood cells. It is potentially curative in over half the patients with CML who receive it, but bone marrow recipients can also die from this aggressive approach, or experience long-term side effects that can be quite debilitating.

Probably the first drug used to treat CML was the poison arsenic, initially given by Thomas Fowler (and henceforth referred to as *Fowler's solution*). In fact, a letter appeared in the British medical journal *Lancet* in 1882 describing the use of arsenic in a patient who likely had CML by no other than a general practitioner named Arthur Conan Doyle, who gained fame (and later, knighthood) for his stories about the detective Sherlock Holmes![13]

More contemporary nontransplant treatments included interferon, an immune therapy that brought about complete remissions, even resulting in a return of normal chromosomes, but in fewer than 10 percent of patients. The side effects to the drug were awful, even leading some patients to commit suicide rather than trying to withstand them. The typical survival for someone with CML was about three and a half years.

Following the development of a "mouse model" of CML, the opportunity arose to start screening existing drugs that had been developed (but were not yet necessarily FDA approved) to see how well these drugs worked to kill CML cells. The drugs were first tried in test tubes that held cells with the Philadelphia chromosome abnormality—essentially, CML cells. If the drugs performed well in test tubes, they were then tried in mice with CML.

One investigator, Brian Druker, who at the time (in the late 1980s) had just finished his training as a hematologist/oncologist at the Dana-Farber Cancer Institute in Boston, dedicated his research to this issue. He focused on CML knowing that because it is a much simpler cancer than other leukemias—a one-hit wonder—the likelihood increased for him to find a single drug to work on the CML cells in a test tube, on CML mice, and eventually on people with CML.[14]

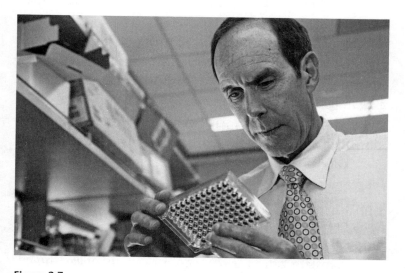

Figure 2.7
Brian Druker, who discovered the drug imatinib and led clinical trials in CML. *Source*: photo courtesy of Oregon Health Sciences University.

So in collaboration with Nick Lyden, who led a drug discovery group at the pharmaceutical company Novartis, Druker started screening drugs and applied for funding to support his research.

And he applied. And he applied.

But funding agencies, including the National Institutes of Health, thought his research proposals were too risky, and likely to fail, so they rejected his grant applications. New laboratory investigators at an academic institution are usually provided some money by the institution to support them and their research for a couple of years, but if that research doesn't take off, they are politely (or sometimes not so politely) asked to leave. Dr. Druker was asked to leave.

He landed at Oregon Health Sciences University in 1993, and he didn't give up. He finally discovered a drug—at the time, called STI-571—that worked incredibly well in CML cells in test tubes, with high kill rates, and in CML mice. It actually was able to rid those mice of their CML entirely, resulting in a rodent remission. The next step was to try the drug in people with CML.

But Novartis, the company that now owned the drug—subsequently called imatinib or referred to by the brand name Gleevec—wasn't so sure. After all, only 6,000 to 9,000 people in the United States were diagnosed with CML each year. Compare that to the almost 20,000 diagnosed with AML, or even the 180,000 people diagnosed with lung cancer, or the more than 200,000 diagnosed with breast cancer or prostate cancer. How would Novartis make enough money to cover the research and development costs?

Dr. Druker appealed to Novartis multiple times, and eventually he prevailed. If the drug worked this well in mice, it had a high likelihood of working well in people and the potential to satisfy a huge public health need. Patients were desperate. At that time, treatment for solid tumors usually lasted for three or four months. CML patients, on the other hand, would have to stay on this drug, daily, for life, meaning they would be paying tens of thousands of dollars per year for the drug, potentially for decades.

You can imagine which one of those arguments Novartis found most compelling.

A clinical trial was initiated in 1998, in which 83 CML patients for whom interferon therapy had not worked or had stopped working were eventually enrolled. The very first patient was a retired railroad engineer from a small town on the coast of Oregon called Tillamook. These folks had few options outside of standard, intravenous chemotherapy, which would only hold their leukemia at bay for a short period of time, if at all.

Something special happened.

Within just a few months, the blood counts of 98 percent of these people, for the first time (for some) in years, returned to being normal. In almost one-third, their Philadelphia chromosome was eradicated, meaning the drug worked at such a deep level that the abnormal genetics driving the disease were corrected. These once-dying patients got out of bed, went dancing or on hikes, even did yoga. And 96 percent of those patients who achieved normal blood counts maintained those normal blood counts a year later. And counting.[15]

When the results of this study were reported, CML patients and their doctors from around the world fell over themselves trying to get access to imatinib. Other CML studies were initiated, enrolling 1,000 patients at 27 medical centers in six countries within just six to nine months.

Dr. Druker had told the drug company that people were desperate. And in May 2001, the US FDA listened and approved imatinib for the treatment of CML. The confirmatory, Phase 3 study, reported in March 2003, randomized over 1,100 CML patients to receive imatinib or interferon combined with cytarabine (the chemotherapy we suggested for treating David Sweeney's AML). The results were equally dramatic: After a year and a half of follow-up, 95 percent of patients treated with imatinib had normalization of their blood counts, compared to 55 percent of those treated with interferon and cytarabine; 85 percent had some degree of eradication of their Philadelphia chromosome with imatinib, compared to 22 percent with interferon and cytarabine. And side effects were much, much more tolerable. Unequivocally, imatinib had changed forever the treatment of CML.[16]

But then something really special happened.

After more than a decade of follow-up, it was found that those patients treated with imatinib on the randomized study had a life span that was about the same as age-matched controls without a CML diagnosis.[17]

As if they never had leukemia to start with.

Since the early 2000s we have seen the development of a second- and even third-generation of drugs that also can eradicate the Philadelphia chromosome (and indeed, are better at doing so than imatinib), and which can be used to treat people for whom imatinib didn't work. The drugs have been so successful that bone marrow transplant for CML is only used now as a last resort, when in rare cases all of these drugs have failed.

"We would recommend a pill called imatinib, also known as Gleevec," I told Ms. Badway. I discussed with her the chances that it would work, the side effects, and how her blood counts would change over the next few weeks. I paused, about to raise the most difficult issue about her treatment, but she beat me to it.

"How will it affect the baby?" She started rubbing her belly again as she asked the question.

I exhaled a while before giving her an answer that was not straightforward. "I don't know whether this is reassuring to you or not, but there are actually some case reports of people with CML who have either been pregnant at the time of their diagnosis, like you, or got pregnant while being treated for CML. So you're not alone.

She smiled at me wryly. Some consolation, but she'd rather not be a member of this elite club.

"If you read therapy guidelines from CML experts on treating pregnant women, they recommend interferon because it does not cross the placenta, and thus won't affect the baby. But it also doesn't treat the CML nearly as well as imatinib."

She nodded, listening, still rubbing her belly as if she were reassuring the baby, *it's okay, I'll keep you safe.*

"To be honest, one problem with the writers of such guidelines is that they tend to be extra conservative, and don't always provide the best basis for their recommendations."

"Why's that?" she asked.

"Well, I think it's because they don't want to suggest a treatment that doesn't fall in line with what everyone else recommends, for one. And perhaps because they don't want to be named in a lawsuit if a doctor somewhere in the world uses the recommended treatment, and a patient has a complication."

Rachel was listening intently to this backstory behind the guidelines, which she was probably using to prepare for her hematology boards.

"So, our leukemia group reviewed the guidelines, the case reports of pregnant women treated with imatinib for CML, and case reports of pregnant women treated with interferon. And it turns out the rates of birth defects, or of lost pregnancies, was the same for either drug."

"Really?" Rachel asked, incredulous. "What about for other tyrosine kinase inhibitors?" She referred to the class of drugs, similar to imatinib and developed subsequently, that treated CML even better than imatinib.

"There aren't as many reports about those drugs being used in pregnancy, because they haven't been on the market for as long, and because pregnant women are almost uniformly excluded from clinical trials of new cancer drugs. That's one reason we have to rely on case reports to determine what is potentially safe for the baby. That's also why I would recommend imatinib, because at least there has been some experience with its being used in pregnancy."

"So," Ms. Badway said, "bottom line, you're saying I should take the chemo pill and the baby will be okay."

"Given the potential benefit of the imatinib, and the risks, I'm recommending you take the pill. But I can't guarantee you won't have the side effects we discussed, and I can't promise that the baby will not be affected, that he won't have birth defects. From all of those case reports the risk of a birth defect—many of which are minor, but some of which aren't—is about 10 percent."

"And if I don't take the pill?"

"Well, we would try the interferon," I answered.

"And if I don't take anything?" she countered, rubbing, rubbing, calming.

I thought about her question for a few seconds. "That's always an option. I do worry that with your blood counts so abnormal, and the guarantee that they will continue to worsen over the next few months if your leukemia isn't controlled, you'd be at risk of infections and bleeding or forming blood clots, and those could all affect the baby's health too."

She nodded, rubbing, rubbing. "I'd like to think about it before deciding."

"That's exactly what I would do," I told her.

3
A Time for Decisions

And indeed there will be time
For the yellow smoke that slides along the street,
Rubbing its back upon the window panes;
There will be time, there will be time
To prepare a face to meet the faces that you meet . . .
And time yet for a hundred indecisions
And for a hundred visions and revisions.
　　　　—T. S. Eliot, "The Love Song of J. Alfred Prufrock," 1915

Most of the time our patients arrive on a stretcher, by dark of night, wearing another hospital's gown. A phalanx of family members trails the stretcher, along with two emergency medical services technicians from the ambulance that brought our new patient to us. A cloud of shock, disbelief, trepidation, and sadness encircles the lot of them as they check in at the floor's front desk and move en masse to the room where our patient, and scores of family and friends, will spend the next month.

But sometimes our patients arrive with less fanfare. Their registration at the front desk, a quiet formality, masks the seriousness of the diagnosis—and perhaps the depth of their despair at this new reality—which has turned their body into a sinister, unfriendly place.

Later in the afternoon, when Joan Walker arrived, she gave her information to Angela, the floor's hospital unit secretary. Her new patient identification band noting her name, birthdate, medical record number, and unique QR code was now firmly in place on her left wrist. She was wearing jeans with brown leather clogs and a purple fleece jacket. Her best friend, also a surgical nurse, stood by her side and pulled Joan's wheeled luggage behind her. The large black bag had a shock of red yarn tied to the handle, so Joan could identify it easily when it came off the conveyor belt at the airport. As she had packed her clothes earlier in the day, she recalled ruefully that the bag's last trip was to Cancún. This would be no Mexican holiday, though she reminded herself that at least it would be all-inclusive.

"You wait right here, honey, and I'll call your nurse," Angela told her. Joan stood patiently, knowing the drill. Before long, a nurse who appeared to be a little older than Joan came up to her.

"Are you Joan? I'm Jane. It's so nice to meet you." She smiled warmly. Jane wore white pants and a white top, with white clogs. Her pockets were filled with pens, syringes, tape, alcohol swabs, and gauze pads—the trappings of a nurse who had been doing her job (and doing it extraordinarily well) for 25 years. Her hair was a reddish brown, and she sported gold-rimmed glasses. "Crazy Janey," I called her, after the subject of Bruce Springsteen's "Spirit in the Night." But there was nothing crazy about Janey's gut feelings when it came to her patients. You better believe that when Janey worried about a patient, I worried about a patient and directed the residents to check on that person more frequently. When Janey wondered if we should adjust a medication, I adjusted the medication. And when Janey told me she felt someone was coming out of the woods after being ill for days, I would start to breathe easier.

"I hear you're a nurse down in Wooster." She grasped Joan's elbow and held onto it, both reassuring and steadying her, and held her gaze for a few seconds. That look said: "We're both nurses. You should be the one escorting a patient to her room, not the one wearing the wristband. I'm going to help you get through this."

Joan just nodded, her eyes misty, acknowledging the enormity of that moment, the awful irony, when caregiver becomes cared for.

It's happened to all of us in healthcare, though in varying degrees of seriousness.[1]

A few years back, I was cycling on my road bike, training for a bicycle ride that raises money for our cancer center. As I headed down a steep hill, my bike started going pretty quickly: 20 miles per hour . . . 25 . . . 30 . . . 35 . . . when all of a sudden I hit a slick patch on the newly paved road and, as if pushed by some vengeful god, my bike slipped away from under me.

Slam! I hit the pavement so hard it took my breath away, with no time to even brace myself. The pain in my side was extreme, but I had the wherewithal to realize that at least I was conscious and able to feel pain. I also remembered that I was in the middle of the road and stood up so I wouldn't get hit in the traffic.

That's when the pain went from extreme to blinding, as I felt broken rib scrape against nearby broken rib. It wasn't until later that I realized the distant, disembodied cry I heard was coming from me. I called my wife and asked her to pick me up, probably in some show of bravado that I really wasn't battered enough to require an ambulance—which of course I did.

When my wife arrived, it took me a couple of minutes to figure out how I would fold myself into the passenger seat of her car. She drove to the nearby community hospital within our health system and dropped me off by the ER doors as she went to park. I clip-clopped in my biking shoes up to the triage desk and gave a breathless greeting to the nurse there.

"Hello there," she answered. "And what happened to you?" she asked, scanning my torn cycling jersey, bloody shoulder and leg, and awkward stance.

"I was biking . . ." breath, breath, ". . . and the bike slipped . . ." breath, breath, ". . . and I fell."

"Ouch. Well, sit down in this chair so I can get your vital signs." She gestured toward a blue plastic chair by her desk. I looked at her uncertainly.

"I don't think . . ." breath, breath, ". . . I can sit."

She looked at me quizzically and walked around the desk to stand next to me. "How fast were you going on this bike?" she asked.

"About 30 . . ." breath, breath, ". . . maybe 35 miles per hour."

She shook her head pityingly and took hold of my elbow, just as Janey had done with Joan. "Oh honey, come walk with me to the other side of the ER. You're a trauma."

She gently led me away from the minor and major medical portion of the ER, never letting go of my arm. When we reached one of the trauma bays, she stopped.

"Now, I'm going to have to call a code for you, and a lot of people are going to come running down here when I do. Why don't I help you off with your clothes, because otherwise they're going to cut them off with trauma scissors." Her kindness was in such contrast to the brutality of the crash, to the unforgiving pain I was feeling, it brought me to tears. Just like Joan.

I nodded my agreement, and she pulled off my shoes, biking pants, and what was left of my shirt, and slipped my arms through the hospital gown sleeves. My transformation was complete—I had become a patient. She eased me on to the stretcher, and chaos erupted as people ran into the bay.

It's at this point that, as a doctor-cum-patient, I tried to make the calculation of whether or not to tell the healthcare workers now tending to me that I was "in the biz." On the plus side, I might be treated like a VIP. On the minus side, I might be treated like a VIP.

Having VIP status in a hospital is not all it's cracked up to be. True, these patients do get to occupy nicer rooms on quieter floors, closer in appearance to a fancy hotel. Which sounds great, except these floors are not disease-specific, and the nurses, doctors, and pharmacists who provide the care may not be specialized in the illness that required the hospitalization.

Doctors and nurses who care for someone labeled "VIP," especially when that VIP is also a medical professional, tend to get more nervous because the number of people scrutinizing their every move will probably be greater than on average. As a result, the likelihood increases that mistakes will be made. The number of consultants involved also increases with efforts to avoid those mistakes, as do the numbers of laboratory and radiology tests.

When I was an intern, I cared for a famous infectious disease specialist who, ironically, had developed an infection requiring intravenous antibiotics. I quickly wrote the order, so he wouldn't have to wait to be treated—but the dose I wrote was twice what was standard. He was the one who caught the mistake just as the antibiotic was being hung by his bed. I slowly walked into his room, tail between my legs, ready to be chewed out for my carelessness. He just laughed, and generously said that he assumed I had tried the higher dose based on a recent study.

So now, having to make a quick decision, I decided to keep it on the down low that I was a doctor. Which lasted for all of about 10 minutes, by which point the nurse had noticed the Fitbit I was wearing to track my activity—the same Fitbit worn by other employees in our health system, so we could qualify for discounts on our health insurance. Sure enough, after X-rays confirmed multiple broken ribs and a pneumothorax (which explained my breathlessness), I was given a private room, visited by a bevy of consultants, and underwent a lot of tests.

On the one hand I appreciated the attention. But I wondered how much of my care was ordinary, and how much extraordinary. It also quickly became apparent how awkward it would be to refuse the recommendations of those in my profession. I didn't want to be known as a "difficult patient" or an "ungrateful colleague."

On the other hand, in situations where my workplace status wasn't known, how enlightening to view the hospital from a patient's perspective. When the transport guy (who must have been popular) wheeled me down to the radiology department the following morning, a Monday, multiple hospital employees stopped him to chat about their weekends. The aroma from the Starbucks cup each of them gripped was robust, and in stark contrast to the anemic cup of brown liquid that had graced my hospital tray just minutes earlier. I tried to look them in the eye and nod a hello, as I would have at my own hospital. I had learned to do that when I moved to the Midwest (where lack of such greetings are associated with anger) from the East Coast (where such regular greetings to strangers might have earned me a reputation of being needy or even unhinged). But I was ignored, just an object on a wheelchair. I vowed that none of my own patients would ever feel so marginalized, so like an outsider, when their illness prevented them from participating in the normal interactions enjoyed by those caring for them.

Janey walked Joan into her room to do intake and get her settled, and Rachel followed them soon after, a bone marrow biopsy kit in her hands. Great—the sooner the biopsy is completed, and a bone marrow sample makes it down to Karl, the sooner we can have a diagnosis and get started on treatment.

Why do we rush people to make decisions about treatment for acute leukemia, often within a day or two of their diagnosis? At first blush, it seems unfair. After all, a woman who eventually is diagnosed with breast cancer that requires chemotherapy may have weeks to consider her options: from the moment she first feels a breast lump while taking a shower; to the time it takes to schedule an appointment with her primary care physician, who confirms that a worrisome lump is present; to the next step of undergoing a confirmatory mammogram or ultrasound; to scheduling a surgical biopsy; to waiting for the pathology results to return; to finally meeting with an oncologist to discuss medical, radiation, and/or surgical treatments.

Unlike breast cancer though, leukemia profoundly affects not only the platelets, and thus the body's ability to stop bleeding, but also the immune system, leaving a person susceptible to life-threatening infections. While Joan had a white blood cell count of 154,000, most of those were probably blasts—the kindergarten cells—and it was really remarkable that she hadn't already caught a devastating cold.

But the clock was ticking. At any moment she could contract an infection that would run rampant through her defenseless body, or she could all of a sudden start to bleed internally. We needed to stop this malignant golem before it killed her.

Theoretically, then, it makes sense to diagnose and treat acute leukemia rapidly. But is there a way to prove it? Along with colleagues at the MD Anderson Cancer Center in Texas, my Cleveland Clinic colleagues and I examined over 1,300 people diagnosed with AML at both of our institutions over a 10-year period.[2] Everyone was treated with an intensive chemotherapy regimen, similar to what I described to David and Betty Sweeney. We measured the time from when a leukemia diagnosis was made to when chemotherapy was started, to see if delays in starting treatment mattered.

What we found was fascinating.

For younger adults, defined in the study as ages 17 to 59 years, treatment delays mattered—a lot. Longer times from diagnosis to starting therapy were significantly associated with a lower chance of entering a remission, and a lower survival rate. With every day that passed, the chance that we could successfully treat a person's leukemia diminished substantially—by almost 10 percent going from a one-day delay to a five-day delay. That's the reason Rachel trailed Joan and Janey into the room to perform Joan's bone marrow biopsy.

But for adults 60 years and older, delays didn't significantly impact remission rates or survival. We hypothesized that older adults with AML did better with delays because, for many, their leukemia evolved from a previous bone marrow disorder like myelodysplastic syndromes, which we suspected in David. Rather than a dramatic change that caused leukemia to grow and cause symptoms, as commonly occurs

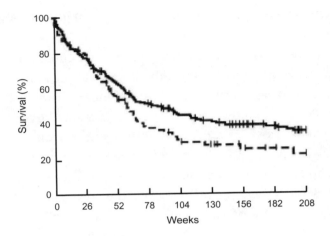

Figure 3.1
Survival is worse for younger AML patients whose treatment is delayed more than five days (the bottom, hashed line) from their diagnosis.

in younger adults, for older folks the leukemia was more of a slippery slide from a previous condition that may have existed for months or even years, and was therefore not as life threatening.

Still, we didn't draw an arbitrary line in the sand at age 60 for whether we would hustle to start therapy or not. For some older adults, the time from diagnosis to starting chemotherapy did matter, if not biologically, certainly psychologically.

I walked over to David's room to see how he was doing. He was still lying in bed, watching the news on the small, flat-screen TV hanging on the wall. I watched him for a minute from the hallway. He held the remote in mid air, as if about to change the channel, but he didn't click it. He was watching, but not watching, distracted, his mind elsewhere. Betty sat in the same chair she had occupied earlier, a cross-word puzzle book open on the bedside table, which she had pulled in front of her. She was using the small golf pencil the hospital provided to every patient to take notes and fill out menu choices. I knocked softly at the open door before entering. They both looked up.

"Anything exciting going on in the world today?" I asked him.

David smiled a bit and shrugged his shoulders. "Oh, you know, crime and politics," he said, vaguely. Betty put her book down.

"And Ohio State football," I offered. "You think they're headed to the National Championship?"

This time Betty smiled. "We put both of our children through Ohio State. They get alumni tickets to the games. In fact, we're planning on going to the Horseshoe in a couple of weeks." A look of uncertainty flickered across her face as she realized mid-sentence that David's future, their future, and the chances that he would be making it to the stadium in two weeks were slim.

"About that," I said, as I sat in a chair by David's bed. "Have you made any decisions about your leukemia?"

"We've talked about it." He glanced over to Betty, who was staring at him, nodding her head faintly. "And I'm not sure it's worth going through all of this, with the aggressive therapy, being cooped up in the hospital and away from family, getting sick, maybe even dying, for such a low chance of being cured. I'd rather take the low-dose stuff and sleep in my own bed every night."

I turned to Betty. "How do you feel about his decision?"

"I'll support whatever he wants to do," she said bravely. David reached over to hold her hand. As she started to cry, he did, too. I grabbed the tissue box from the window seat and brought it to them. I was about to sit back down when a man and woman, both a decade or so younger than me, entered the room. They wore leather jackets, his brown and hers black. She sported an Ohio State scarf around her neck. David introduced them as Eric and Susan, his and Betty's children.

"Can you explain to them what's going on with David?" Betty asked me. Eric walked over by his mom and leaned against the window seat. Susan sat on the bed by her dad.

I reviewed much of what I discussed earlier in the day about David's diagnosis and treatment options, along with the chances the therapies would work. As I spoke, Susan gave her dad quick glances, checking to see how he reacted to my description. They seemed close. When I finished talking, Eric piped up.

"When can you get started on the hospital chemo?" he asked.

David cleared his throat. "I'm not sure I want to go that route. I'm thinking of taking the other drug that I can get in the doctor's clinic."

Eric popped up from the window seat. "Dad, you can't do that!" he exclaimed. "Your only chance of beating this is by getting the high-dose chemo. The doctor says it has a good chance of working. You can't just give up like this."

"He's not giving up," Betty countered. "And the doctor said he only had a 50/50 shot with that chemo. And he could die getting it."

"Well, he'll die if he doesn't get it," Eric answered, and crossed his arms.

"Dad's thought about this carefully, Eric," Betty said. "He doesn't want to be cooped up in the hospital for a month."

"If I'm going to die, I want to die in my own bed," David said quietly.

Susan had placed her hand on David's leg and was looking at him intently. "Daddy, we want you around," she said. "I'm not ready to let you go." She started crying, and David's face collapsed into tears.

"Why don't you all talk this over a bit and I can come back," I said, unnecessarily. At that moment, I was the least important person in the room.

How people make decisions about treating their cancers is complicated. One reason is that both patients—and doctors—exaggerate the benefits of interventions and minimize the harms. In one systematic review of 35 studies that enrolled over 27,000 patients, most participants overestimated benefit for 65 percent of outcomes, and underestimated harm for 67 percent.[3] These studies included interventions like mammography or colonoscopy screening for breast and colon cancer, or mastectomy to prevent breast cancer.

Doctors don't fare much better. In another systematic review of 48 studies that included more than 13,000 clinicians, some of which asked about benefits of cancer screening or risks of cancer from other interventions such as radiation exposure associated with CT scans, more than half the participants overestimated benefits, and underestimated harm, for almost one-third of outcomes.[4] The authors of these studies speculated that such unrealistic optimism stems from core psychological needs such as hope, safety, a sense of control, the need for action, and even reassurance that the right decision has been made. Add to this the clinicians' conviction that they need to act when tragedy strikes—tragedy, in this case, being cancer.

One of my favorite sayings in medicine is "Don't just do something—stand there!" The hardest decision I ever have to make is to not test or treat a patient, or to be comfortable offering a "no therapy" option to someone like David Sweeney, and to be genuinely supportive if that's the route the patient decides to go.

After all, I haven't lived the same life David has. Thus, I can't know what factors he uses to weigh risks and benefits or how to assess the influence of people he holds dear in his life.

I once took care of an Amish man, from a town not too far from where Joan lived, whose white beard made him look much older than his 50 years. Like David, he had acute leukemia, and I had a discussion about treatment options with him similar to the one I had with David and Betty. The difference, because of his younger age, was in the estimates

I gave him for going into a remission (about 20 percent higher), death from the treatment (about 10 percent lower), and chance of being cured (about 30 percent higher).

"What if I chose to leave the hospital without treatment and go back home?" he asked me.

Given his age, I was a bit surprised that he wanted to consider this option.

He explained to me that he was a deacon in his community and was privy to the hospital bills that resulted when other members had become ill. Many Amish don't have private insurance, but as a community they pool their resources to pay the bills. He didn't want to cripple others financially to pay for his healthcare.

As he put it, "This world is not my final destiny, anyway."[5]

Another patient, a man in his 60s, had a leukemia that kept returning, despite our best efforts at containing it. He and his wife made the regular hour-and-a-half drive to my clinic in their aging car, which itself had become less and less dependable. When I broached the topic of another round of therapy, a pill that would not be covered entirely by his insurance, I also had to discuss the $5,000 monthly out-of-pocket price tag. This, too, had become part of my informed consent process: risks, benefits, alternatives, and financial toxicity. He declined the treatment in favor of hospice.

As he put it, "I won't bankrupt my family for a month or two more time. I have to leave them something."[6]

People also make decisions to take chemotherapy given chances that I, personally, would have thought to be too against their favor to be worthwhile. These are the gamblers, the folks who "chase the tails" of survival curves, meaning the handful of people in clinical trials who were cured despite the long-shot odds.

In a study that I led when I was still in my training fellowship in Boston, I approached older adults, like David, who were just given a diagnosis of acute leukemia.[7] My colleagues and I asked them a series of questions about their quality of life—in other words, how much the leukemia was causing them to feel fatigued, depressed, or worried—and questions about how they made the decision to receive the aggressive, inpatient chemotherapy, or the lower-dose, outpatient option.

We found that physical functioning among patients was more than one-and-a-half standard deviations below the general population (about 30 percent worse) and that 35 percent of patients were depressed—numbers far worse than we would have guessed. The physical functioning scores deteriorated significantly for hospitalized patients after they started the high-dose chemotherapy, but then rebounded as soon as they were discharged back home, and continued to improve over months for those who entered a remission. Among people who chose to receive therapy as an outpatient, where remission rates were less than half of the aggressive inpatient therapy, physical functioning worsened at a slower pace, but never rebounded like it did for those hospitalized. Depression continued to worsen in this group also, reaching a peak of almost 50 percent six weeks after the first survey.

These findings led us to beef up our psychosocial supports for our patients, and to be deliberate in asking questions that touched on their emotions, rather than just their blood counts. Assessing sadness or despondency has become another vital sign.

When we asked people how they made decisions, the results surprised us even more. Almost two-thirds of patients told us that they had not been offered treatment options other than the one they chose—despite conversations taking place that were almost identical to the one I had with David and Betty, in which three options (aggressive chemotherapy, low-dose chemotherapy, or supportive care [no chemotherapy]) were discussed.

Those choosing the aggressive chemotherapy were more likely than those choosing the low-dose outpatient treatment (74 percent versus 47 percent) to say their decision was influenced by their doctor. Yet, when we asked the same patients what they estimated their chance of cure to be, 74 percent reported it to be >50 percent—despite 89 percent of their doctors having communicated the chance of being cured as being <10 percent, as I had to David. This even occurred when the survey questions were administered to the patients and to their doctors just a few minutes after the discussion about risks and benefits of chemotherapy took place.

Why did this happen?

It may be that all the talk about how leukemia arose, how to treat it, the side effects of treatment, the hospital stay, the likelihood the chemotherapy would work, and survival estimates was simply an information overload. In other words, my colleagues and I may be poor communicators in the sense that we don't convey information in a way that people can process or remember it.

In a study conducted at the Dana-Farber Cancer Institute in Boston and the Fred Hutchinson Cancer Research Center in Seattle, interactions between 40 hematologist/oncologists and more than 230 patients over a four-year period were audio recorded, and the transcripts analyzed.[8] The average duration of each interaction was almost 70 minutes.

In one analysis of this study, the most common technique doctors used in communicating with patients was called "broadcasting": a pattern of lengthy physician monologues on disease mechanisms and history, treatment options, or prognostic information, often lasting for 10 minutes or longer![9] Doctors did not invite interruptions. Some used deferential language (referring to how "some patients" would make a treatment decision, or telling patients "you need to figure out" the right course of action), while others were directive ("I would vote for the first treatment option"). The favored style of communication was one that invited patient participation by using open-ended questions ("What have you been told about treatment for your cancer?").

People who choose to receive aggressive chemotherapy may choose to remember the best odds, or exaggerate those odds, to bolster the justification for their decision. Or, some may enter a type of adaptive denial to cope with both their diagnosis and the long-shot odds of chemotherapy curing them. A more positive spin to this coping mechanism is to call it optimism, or hope—both of which have been associated with better outcomes among cancer patients. For example, one study showed better early survival among 300 patients undergoing bone marrow transplant, and another study showed improved five-year survival rates for 530 non-pessimistic people with lung cancer.[10]

If that's the case, I hope to experience the same adaptive denial if I'm diagnosed with an illness that is potentially terminal.

A separate study in 260 patients undergoing a bone marrow transplant found that those with higher-risk cancers—meaning that their expected survival following the transplant was lower—tended to be much more optimistic about their chances than their doctors. Those with a likely favorable outcome following the transplant tended to have expectations that were more concordant with what their doctors estimated.[11]

For the study I led during my training, it sometimes took 30 minutes or more to administer the survey questions depending on how many times a patient and I got interrupted. Inevitably, a patient or family member would stop me before I left the hospital room.

"Why is somebody like you asking me all of these questions?" they wanted to know.

I would adjust my white coat, a little bit confused. "What do you mean?"

"You're a doctor, don't you have more important things to do?"

More important than trying to understand what it feels like to have leukemia, and how my patients make decisions about their future? I couldn't imagine what that could be.

I walked over to Joan's room just as Rachel was leaving.

"How'd it go?" I asked Rachel, who was peeling off a protective paper gown for the second time that day.

"Good. I didn't feel a thing," she wisecracked. "Actually, it did go well, but she kept bleeding from the puncture site for a while. I had to hold pressure on it for about 20 minutes, and even then it was still oozing. So I put a pressure dressing on the site and asked Ms. Walker to lie flat for an hour."

"Do you think it bled more than usual?" I asked. She nodded. "Can you send some coags?"

"Way ahead of you, boss. They're cooking," she answered. Rachel was the type of fellow who was so smart that I had to work to find some esoteric fact about our patients I could teach her.

Coags, short for coagulation labs, are a group of tests that measure the ability of the blood to form clots. It's bad enough that someone has a diagnosis of acute leukemia, which usually causes the platelet count to be low, predisposing that person to bleeding. We already knew that was the situation with Joan. It's even worse when the blood's ability to coagulate the sparse numbers of platelets is impaired, a condition called disseminated intravascular coagulopathy, or DIC. DIC can arise as a side effect of certain types of leukemias, or it can be triggered by a serious infection. It can be devastating, as DIC can lead to either life-threatening bleeding, or to the formation of blood clots that could be equally dire.

I knocked on Joan's open door gently. She was lying flat in bed, now wearing the Diane von Furstenberg duds. There was some blood staining her sheets. Her eyes were shut, and her friend had left the room, probably ushered out by Janey when Rachel performed the bone marrow biopsy. While we loved having friends and family members around frequently to support our patients and help them get through the ordeal of treatment, we have learned from past experiences that once one of us brandishes that absurdly long needle for the biopsy, some people faint. And then we have two patients, instead of one. That situation is one I call an IGBO—I Got Burned Once.

"Hey," I said softly. She opened her eyes and looked over to me. Rachel followed me in.

"Hey," she answered, almost reluctantly, as if she didn't want this next stage of her life to begin yet.

"Okay for me to sit down?" I asked, gesturing to her bed. She nodded, and I introduced myself. "You know why you're here?" She nodded again.

"I sure would have liked to be meeting you in the outpatient clinic in Wooster," I offered. She grimaced. "I hear you're a surgical nurse. You have a really good group there. Your patients are lucky to have you."

"Yeah, they're the best," she agreed.

"We're pretty concerned that you have leukemia," I said. "What do you know about it?"

"Only that anyone I've taken care of with leukemia in the ICU hasn't done too well," She replied. "Especially the bone marrow transplant patients."

"It's true, our patients have to be pretty sick to make it to the ICU, and once they get there, many don't make it out. But some do. And my goal is to keep you out of the ICU as we get rid of this leukemia," I told her. She was quiet, tearing up a bit.

In many hospitals, there is a bias that cancer patients shouldn't be admitted to intensive care units, the perception being that they never make it out of them alive. A few years before I treated Joan, we had decided to study this phenomenon to see if it was true. We followed 90 patients with acute leukemia who were admitted to our intensive care unit so we could evaluate how they did.[12] Approximately one-third improved enough during their ICU stay to continue receiving aggressive therapy for their leukemia; most of them were eventually discharged from the hospital back home. Those who did not need to be placed on a mechanical ventilator and did not require medicines (called *pressors*) to raise a low blood pressure had the best outcome of all, with over half surviving the hospitalization. The main take-home message from the study was that people with acute leukemia fared no worse than those with other serious medical conditions who were admitted to the ICUs at the same time. There was no basis for the bias.

Joan's friend walked into the room with an older woman who came straight over to the bed to give Joan a hug. Joan introduced her to me as her sister Connie. I could see the resemblance, in the eyes and the edges of their mouths. She also introduced her nurse friend Patty.

"Connie's 15 years older than me," Joan said. "I was planned, she was the accident." I laughed as Joan and Connie smiled at what I'm sure was a well-tread joke, repeated over years. Joan asked me to explain what was going on to Connie and her friend, and by association to her too.

I reviewed a lot of the same facts that I had discussed earlier in the day with David and Betty and their children. I shifted some of the outcome estimates given Joan's younger age, quoting a 70 percent chance of entering a remission, a risk of dying less than 10 percent, and a chance of being alive in five years of approximately one-third. No one took notes, but everyone listened attentively.

"I'm confused," Connie said. "If Joan has a 70 percent chance of a remission, why does that drop to 30 percent five years from now. Doesn't remission means she's cured?"

I reflected back to the study we conducted when I was in my training, and wondered whether the people I surveyed really overestimated their chances of being cured, or were conflating remission estimates with cure. Either way, the onus was on me to do a better job explaining the critical difference.

"We can only detect cancer in the body when you have 10 billion cancer cells. Below that amount, we might not even notice anything abnormal on a CT scan for a solid tumor like lung cancer, or see anything abnormal in blood counts for hematologic cancers like leukemia."

"So right now, Joan has more than 10 billion leukemia cells in her body," Patty commented, her eyes widening at the enormity of the number. A statement, not a question.

I nodded, looking at Joan. "You do. When we give you this first round of chemotherapy, our goal is to reduce that number 1,000-fold or 10,000-fold—by three or four logarithms, down to maybe 10 million cells. If we're successful, we'll know it because we'll perform another bone marrow biopsy on you and we won't be able to see any of the leukemia cells."

"Even with 10 million of them still floating around?" Patty asked.

"That's right," I answered. "Remission means we can't see any of the leukemia using a microscope to view a section of the bone marrow, with the blood counts mostly recovered back to normal. Remission is a wonderful thing. It's the first step toward being cured. But it doesn't mean the leukemia's gone."

"So you have to give more chemo after that, to get rid of what's left over," Joan said.

I nodded again. "Yup. That's what we call *post-remission* therapy. It's mainly done in the outpatient clinic. Every time we give another cycle of chemo, we hopefully reduce the number of leukemia cells another 100- to 1,000-fold. So, from 10 million cells to 100,000, and then from 100,000 to 1,000, and so on. Eventually, there is such a low level of leukemia remaining that, hopefully, your immune system can gobble up the rest."

"And then she's cured," Patty said. I agreed. "Even at a genetic level?"

I hesitated. "You've been doing some reading?" I asked Patty.

She nodded. "What I could on the drive up here."

She seemed like a great friend, and a super advocate for Joan. I hoped I was lucky enough to have someone like Patty with me if I ever had a serious illness.

"Leukemia starts when something goes wrong in the genetic machinery of the bone marrow cells—the blueprints for the cell." I clarified that most of the time these weren't genes that were passed down to children. "When we talk about remission, we said that we couldn't see any leukemia cells as hard as we look. Sometimes, though, we can still detect the abnormal genes. This is a condition we call *minimal residual disease* with a *morphologic* remission—we can't see the leukemia cells, but we know they're still there because the bad genes are lurking. We can sometimes use that information to our advantage—it means there's a greater likelihood the leukemia will return despite the traditional remission, and we might intensify the therapy we use in the future, even recommending a bone marrow transplant. So we'll look for any of these genetic abnormalities to see if we can follow their levels over time."

"Can you treat any of the genetic abnormalities?" Patty asked.

"We can," I answered. "There are a couple that have been discovered in the past few years that are associated with AML. One, called *FLT3*, can be targeted with a drug that was just approved in 2017. People who received the drug, along with chemotherapy, lived longer than those who were just treated with the chemo. Another, called *IDH2*, can be treated with a pill."

Patty and Joan were rapt with attention. Connie stared at Joan, her eyes unfocused, probably still shell-shocked that her younger sister had a life-threatening diagnosis.

I hesitated before I continued, wanting them to absorb what I had just said but not wanting to raise their hopes prematurely with what I had to say next. I gestured to Rachel.

"Rachel tells me that you had some bleeding after she performed the biopsy."

Joan glanced quickly at Rachel, then back to address me. "I guess so. The young doctor did a good job with the needle, but could use a little work on her pressure dressings," Joan joked.

"Hey, hey, they haven't taught us that in fellowship yet!" Rachel answered, joining the repartee. "The bleeding stopped, didn't it?"

"Doctor, eventually all bleeding stops," Joan quipped. She was a riot.

"Great point!" I laughed. "But in all seriousness, while the bleeding could have occurred with your low platelet count, it also may mean you have some DIC."

"That's not good," Joan answered, alarm now replacing her previous, mischievous look. "When my patients develop DIC, they almost never make it out of the hospital alive."

"Well, maybe. But paradoxically it may actually be an encouraging sign. DIC can occur with any type of leukemia,

but it occurs more frequently with one subtype, acute promyelocytic leukemia, or APL, which has a really good prognosis. We were just talking about the genetics of leukemia.
This one is associated with abnormalities of chromosomes
15 and 17." A translocation, like with *BCR-ABL* in Ms. Badway's chronic myeloid leukemia. "We're sending tests both
to see if you have DIC, and to check if you have this type of
leukemia. I should know more later today about the DIC,
and by tomorrow about the leukemia."

"We'll keep our fingers crossed," Patty responded.

"Yes," Connie added, looking at Rachel and me. "Fingers
and toes."

If you're playing the parlor game "What kind of leukemia
would I want to get?" the answer of course, is "none." But if
forced to claim one, my answer would be CML. If the follow-
up question asks which kind of *acute* leukemia would I want
to get, the answer would be acute promyelocytic leukemia
or APL.

And it goes without saying, that if these are the types of
parlor games you're playing, you need to get out more often.

APL used to be a death sentence. It was first described
in 1957 by a Norwegian hematologist, L. K. Hillestad, who
wrote that its "most outstanding feature was its very rapidly
downhill course of few weeks' duration, a white blood cell
dominated by promyelocytes and severe bleeding."[13] The
severe bleeding was brought about by the DIC we suspected
in Joan. Promyelocytes, like blasts, are immature white blood
cells doomed to an eternal childhood by the translocation

of chromosomes 15 and 17, which blocks the cells from becoming a functional immune system. Janet Rowley at the University of Chicago—the same Janet Rowley who discovered the *BCR-ABL* translocation in CML—identified this genetic basis for the leukemia.[14] Her work on the genetics of leukemia earned her a Lasker Award in 1998 and a Presidential Medal of Freedom award in 2009.

In APL, the promyelocytes have a peculiar appearance. Their interiors are filled with azure-colored granules, which will sometimes stick together to form rods. These are called "Auer" rods, after the physiologist John Auer, who described them in 1906 in a 21-year-old patient suffering from nosebleeds, although Thomas McCrae, a physician at Johns

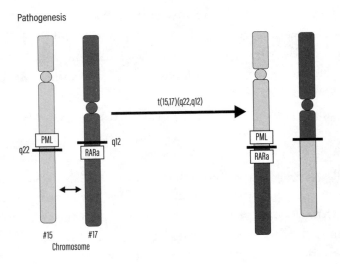

Figure 3.2

The translocation of chromosomes 15 and 17 creating the PML-RAR alpha (RARa) chromosome that causes acute promyelocytic leukemia.

Hopkins, had described them also, a year earlier. Auer rods resemble bunches of sticks—known as faggots—a linchpin in making the diagnosis.[15]

It wasn't until the early 1970s that any chemotherapy was reported to successfully mitigate this dismal outcome. That chemotherapy was daunorubicin (the same drug we discussed with the Sweeneys), which improved remission rates in 80 patients with APL treated at Hôpital Saint-Louis, in Paris, from 13 percent to 57 percent.[16]

Meanwhile, in the lab, a couple of groups of scientists were discovering that leukemia cells could be triggered to undergo maturation (toward becoming functional white blood cells) with certain agents, including retinoic acid.

The next major breakthrough in treating APL came in the mid to late 1980s. Zhen-Yi Wang, a doctor in China, gave a pill called all-*trans* retinoic acid (ATRA) to a five-year-old girl with APL whose disease did not go into remission after treatment with daunorubicin.[17]

This was nothing more than a vitamin A derivative. She went from a condition that, in Wang's words, was "hopeless" to a remission, and eventually was cured. He then reported the results of his experience treating 24 patients with APL (some of whom had disease recurrence after previously being treated with chemotherapy) at the Rui-Jin Hospital in Shanghai. Remarkably, 23 of his patients achieved a remission—with a vitamin!

And these patients didn't experience the precipitous, life-threatening drop in their blood counts that I had described to the Sweeneys, the necessary evil of standard chemotherapy.

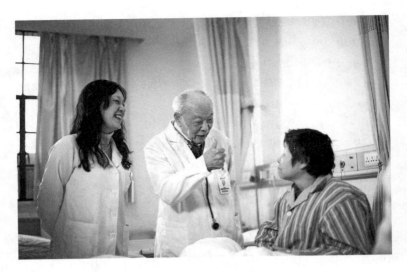

Figure 3.3
Zhen-Yi Wang, the Chinese doctor who first used all-*trans* retinoic acid to treat acute promyelocytic leukemia.

Wang's findings upended the dogma of needing to treat all leukemias with toxic chemotherapy.

As with Brian Druker's research on treatments for CML, though, there were doubters. For starters, the clinical report of the vitamin's efficacy preceded the knowledge about the genetic basis for APL, and how that translocation caused the promyelocytes to freeze at their immature development stage. This finding would subsequently be elucidated in the early 1990s in increments: first with cloning of the translocation of chromosomes 15 and 17 and identification of the relevant genes (subsequently named the retinoic acid receptor alpha [*RARA*] and promyelocytic leukemia [*PML*] genes); next with experiments in cells that mimicked APL and with recapitulation of APL in mice, similar to what George Daley and David Baltimore had done with CML; and finally with research that determined how the translocation caused the promyelocytes to stop maturing.

Another more sinister reason why the report from Wang didn't change medical practice overnight was because some doctors in Western countries simply didn't believe him. Many trained in Western medicine have a longstanding mistrust of Eastern medical practices. Acupuncture for back pain? Herbal remedies for colds? A vitamin that can cure leukemia? Yeah, right!

Some of the explanation for the use of ATRA to treat APL was steeped in Confucian philosophy and its belief in the rehabilitation of criminals. Wang and a former star PhD student of his, Zhu Chen, quote a relevant passage from the *Analects*:

> If you use laws to direct the people, and punishments to control them, they will merely try to evade the laws, and will have no sense of shame. But if by virtue you guide them, and by the rites you control them, there will be a sense of shame and of right.[18]

The disease control model in China was influenced by this ancient philosophy about ways to control society. ATRA caused the criminal bone marrow elements (corrupt promyelocytes) to become stand-up citizens (mature white blood cells). Western doctors, in particular, were more likely to take college courses in biochemistry than near-Eastern philosophy, and probably did not buy in to the theory.

So, unfortunately, the delay in the uptake of ATRA resulted from a pervasive mistrust among Western scientists about the validity of research coming out of China, that continues to this day.

"They lie," I have heard colleagues say, referring to Chinese investigators.

"I just don't believe the results." I have seen this statement among comments from people reviewing Chinese research submissions to Western medical journals—submissions that were subsequently rejected.

Was this suspicion due to language barriers? A cultural divide? Racism? A recognition that Chinese scientists may be under more pressure to show success at any cost? Probably a bit of all four.

Wang and Chen started collaborating with doctors at Hôpital Saint-Louis around the same time (1988) as their publication. When similar results were reported in French patients in 1990, the mighty little vitamin could no longer be ignored.[19] It ushered in a decade of clinical trials that incorporated ATRA into various chemotherapy regimens. Chemotherapy wasn't abandoned, because investigators realized that the remission attained with the ATRA pills alone usually lasted just a few months. But when chemotherapy was combined with ATRA, the treatment approaches packed a one-two punch that led to remissions in about 90 percent of patients, and a cure rate that approached 80 percent.

In fact, unlike with other acute leukemias, for which chemotherapy can either lead to remission, death, or can be ineffective—with a person neither achieving remission nor dying—in APL, treatment regimens incorporating ATRA have a binary outcome: remission or death. And most people who die do so because of bleeding complications, almost uniformly as a consequence of DIC.

The junior resident, John, came up to me and Rachel as we returned to the hallway outside Joan's room. He looked even more disheveled than he had that morning.

"You need to get home buddy, I worry about you," I said to him.

"What, and miss out on all the learning I could be doing here?" He smiled at me, wanly. It sounded like the sort of thing I would say when I was a resident.

"I'm almost done, just tying up some loose ends. The Sweeneys want to speak with you."

"Has he decided about chemotherapy?" I asked.

"I think so," John answered. "There was a pretty heated conversation going on in there earlier. It's calmed down."

I walked over to David's room, with Rachel and John trailing, knocked at his door, and entered. Susan was now sitting in the chair Betty had occupied before, while Eric remained leaning against the window seat, his arms still crossed. David lay in his bed, and Betty was nowhere to be seen.

"Hey everyone," I said. David lifted his hand in greeting, and Susan said "Hi" in a whisper. Her eyes were red from crying. Eric nodded at me. "Have you made a decision about your treatment, or do you have any more questions you'd like to ask?"

"Doc, I'd like to get that high-test chemo you give in the hospital. I'm going to give this thing my best shot," David answered. Susan stared at him intently as he spoke, her eyes unwavering.

"You sure about this?" I asked. "A little while ago you told me you were leaning toward the outpatient chemo. Once we get started with this, it's hard to back away."

Eric shifted from one foot to the other, impatiently. Susan looked down.

"I'm sure," David answered again. "I want to do what's right for everyone. I can make it through the chemo."

"We know you can Dad," Eric echoed.

"Thanks, Daddy," Susan whispered. She took his hand.

"Okay then. You know I'll support whatever you decide is right for you."

"This is what's right," he answered.

"I'll write for the chemo and we'll get it going in an hour or two," I said. Eric exhaled, relieved. "Where's Betty?" I asked. She had been David's ally when he made his initial decision to take the lower-dose chemotherapy.

"She went down to the cafeteria to get a cup of coffee," Susan responded.

"I think she needed some alone time," David added. I could only imagine what an emotional roller coaster this day had been for them all.

Back in the hallway, Rachel shook her head, clearly frustrated.

"It's not right," she said. "He doesn't want to be here. He doesn't want to get the Ara-C and daunorubicin. He only agreed to it because his kids wanted him to be aggressive."

I nodded my head. "Everything you're saying is true Rachel. But let me ask you this: Is it wrong to make a decision about your healthcare because it's in the best interests of your family? For the people you love and who love you?"

David certainly wouldn't be the only one of my patients who chose a more aggressive path to treat leukemia because that's what their children or spouse wanted. In the study we conducted during my training fellowship, we also asked people with leukemia what influenced the treatment decision they eventually made. Most (97 percent) reported that quality of life was more important to them than length of life. A majority (61 percent) said that their doctor influenced their treatment decision, and 30 percent went so far as to say that their doctor (and not they, themselves) made the decision about their medical care. But a group of patients (21 percent) told us that their family influenced their treatment choice. Interestingly, 11 percent admitted that they had seen a friend or family member receive chemotherapy and didn't want any part of it based on what they observed.

I've also cared for people who decided on less aggressive paths because of family considerations. One woman in her late 60s declined inpatient chemotherapy because she had to return home to look after her mother, who was in her 90s.

"She has dementia. She depends on me," my patient told me.

"Do you have any siblings who can help out?" She shook her head. "What about finding a place for her in a long-term care facility?"

She shook her head more vigorously. "No way. I promised her I would take care of her, that I'd never let that happen. And that's what I'm going to do."

A lot of my patients are older, and live their lives bouncing from one medical catastrophe to another, organizing their weeks around their own or their partner's doctors' appointments.[20] Another patient, a man in his 70s with leukemia, was married to a woman who developed colon cancer at the same time. He delayed his treatment so he could care for her while she was getting chemotherapy, and then she delayed a subsequent round of her therapy so she could care for him.

People make sacrifices for each other when it comes to health, just as they do for families and careers. Each of these decisions was the right one to make at that time, for that person.

"I would choose what's best for my health if I had leukemia." Rachel said.

"Fair enough," I responded. "You and I are at different stages of life than Mr. Sweeney, Ms. Badway, or Ms. Walker. Our job is to help them make their own decisions."

The leukemia pharmacist, whose name was Caitlin, walked over to us. Ms. Badway was following her down the hallway.

"Could you sign the order for Ms. Badway's Gleevec?" she asked me.

"You decided to take the pill?" I asked Ms. Badway, as she approached us.

She nodded. "I gotta do whatever I can to fight this leukemia. My health has to come first. I'll feel terrible if the baby gets birth defects, but I'm not going to do him or any of the other kids any favors if I'm not around."

"I understand," I said to her. "I think it's a good decision. Let's get you the pills and you can bust outta here. I'd like to see you in a couple of days in my clinic, and we'll need OB to follow you weekly also."

"You really think it's a good decision?" she asked, stroking her belly gently.

"I wouldn't give you any options that I wouldn't support 100 percent." I answered. "It's a great decision. It's what's best for you."

4
The Purgatory of the Hospital

The caged bird sings
with fearful trill
of the things unknown
but longed for still

—Maya Angelou, "Caged Bird," 1983

I walked down the eight flights of stairs from the leukemia floor to the Skyway, a main drag connecting the sundry buildings of the sprawling Cleveland Clinic hospital complex. From there I would take another hallway leading to the outpatient cancer center, and then some stairs up to my office. On one side, I could stare out north, through the windows, in the direction of Lake Erie and the hospital's semicircular main drive, to the new medical, dental, and nursing school building across Euclid Avenue. On the other side, I looked south at a large parking garage and the basic science research building, which houses laboratories, biomechanical engineering facilities, and even the front offices where the CEO and his staff work. The irony of having caged rodents in the research building, and my following this human habitrail of connections to my own nest, did not escape me.

As was true of the Mayo Clinic, the Cleveland Clinic hospital was born from war. George Washington Crile, MD, organized the American military hospital in Paris in 1915, later leading the US Army Base Hospital #4 in Rouen, France. Prior to serving overseas, Crile was in practice with Frank E. Bunts, MD, and Crile's cousin William Lower, MD; both of them also served in the Rouen hospital. In France the three doctors discussed the creation of a new medical center in Cleveland, where they could continue to practice some of the military surgical procedures they were developing. John Phillips joined them in these discussions and in the eventual founding of the Cleveland Clinic upon their return.[1]

A four-story building, which housed all of the clinic's 60 employees, was dedicated in February 1921. One of the Mayo brothers, William Benson Mayo, delivered the keynote address. The pale, brick edifice still stands today, though its original, large atrium has been turned into two floors. It is also easy to miss: the clinic's footprint quickly expanded after opening with a new hospital building in 1924, and even-newer buildings surround and nearly engulf it now; major expansions in the 1950s, 1980s, and at the close of the last century have necessitated the Daedalus-inspired connectors through which I walk on a daily basis.

But in May 1929, only eight years after opening, the Cleveland Clinic almost came to an end when some nitrocellulose X-ray films ignited in the basement of one of its buildings. Nitrocellulose, the flexible film base first used in products made by the Eastman Kodak Company in 1889, had developed a reputation for being highly flammable and

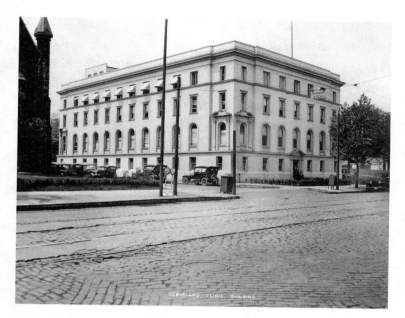

Figure 4.1
The original Cleveland Clinic outpatient building in 1921.

difficult to extinguish with water. The combination of the
fire and toxic fumes from the films quickly spread throughout the hospital, leading to the deaths of 123 people, including patients, employees, visitors, and the hospital founder
John Phillips. Victims were carried by stretcher, or even
slung over the shoulders of volunteers, to be cared for on the
front lawn of the hospital. After relocating temporarily to a
nearby building, the clinic resumed patient care services five
days later, and hasn't closed since.[2]

The cause of the fire, though never precisely determined,
was thought to have been due to a discarded match or cigarette, spontaneous combustion due to heat, or contact with

a light-fixture cord near the films. The legacy of the blaze persists to this day: fire-fighting approaches, hospital procedures, and guidance on the proper storing of hazardous materials nationwide have been revised as a result of the fire, and all 50,000-plus employees at the clinic undergo extensive fire prevention and recognition training when we start our jobs, and we take refresher courses every year.

In 2017, the new Cleveland Clinic Taussig Cancer Center opened, a structure remarkable for its cantilevered glass facade, and for the clean white and gray interior walls interspersed with colorful artworks. If you troll the clinic's Twitter feed frequently enough, you'll see photos showing how the reflective glass of its exterior mirrors the sun and clouds in the sky to evoke a Magritte-like trompe l'oeil. Works featured in the building and on the entire hospital grounds number 6,500 paintings, photographs, sculptures, and mixed media installations or objects. Artists represented include Eva Rothschild, Rana Begum, and Spencer Finch, whose "Trying to Remember the Color of the Sky on That September Morning" is the only work of art to grace the National September 11 Memorial Museum. The Art Program at the clinic adheres to the belief that "fine art is good medicine," in that it "comforts, elevates the spirit, and affirms life and hope."[3]

The Boston-based William Rawn Associates designed the building, its focus on empathy for patients apparent even as the building was going up. Construction workers decorated a ribbon wall, each ribbon commemorating a loved one or family member of their own with cancer.[4] Every day those workers walked by that wall, in their hard hats and bright orange vests, they must have been reminded who would be cared for within the completed structure, and what it was like when, as family member or friend, they sat by the infusion chair as the chemo dripped into a loved one. Before the last steel beam was placed, a bunch of us donned the same hats and vests and, using a silver Sharpie, wrote our names and a message to our patients on a girder. We all had something personal invested in that building, right down to its bones.

Similarly, when the new Dana-Farber Cancer Institute building was erected in Boston in 2016, construction workers there wrote the names of patients on the steel beams after seeing signs held aloft by children with cancer in the windows of the old building across the street. Another reminder of what was at stake within the confines of these spaces.

The newer buildings on campus evoke an antiseptic environment run by professionals, intended to inspire confidence in patients seeking treatment with us. With the new cancer building, I worried that the sterility of the surroundings would instead cause patients to think we were cold and indifferent, more of a business rather than a team of healthcare workers who care deeply about their patients. I was wrong, though—my patients repeatedly told me how much they loved the space, particularly the light streaming through the windows. In fact, when we participated in designing the building, we specified that the windows by the chemotherapy treatment rooms needed to be tinted, as many of the drugs we administer can make people more susceptible to sunburn.

When I am on service—taking care of people in the hospital—my office becomes no more than a closet, a place where I trade an outdoor jacket for a white coat in the morning, and a white coat for an outdoor jacket in the evening. One braces me against the elements of Cleveland weather, the other against bodily fluids. The first evening after meeting Joan and David, I grabbed my fall jacket and headed outside to the fresh air for the first time in 12 hours. As I crossed Carnegie Avenue to the parking garage, I saw the sun dip behind the downtown skyline. It was pretty, and sad at the same time, as my day had been bracketed by the sun's rising and setting.

When I graduated medical school, I came in possession of the first car I ever owned—a late 1980s white Plymouth Turismo, passed down from a grandmother whose vision had so deteriorated that she'd been declared a driving menace. That dinged and dented car lasted for about three months before its transmission essentially exploded, and I had to get a new vehicle, fast.

Interns don't have much in the way of leisure time, so I was only able to "shop around" at a nearby used car lot when I was post-call, having gone approximately 36 hours without any shuteye. In this state of sleep-deprived concupiscence, I decided it would be a great idea to buy a convertible.

In Boston. With winter approaching.

The car, a Honda Del Sol, performed admirably in October. But it fell a bit shy of expectations come February, when its light weight, low clearance, and dicey defroster frequently lost the battle against the heavy New England snow and the frustrated efforts of the Boston Public Works Department. Still, I adored that car, and every day the weather allowed, I would pop off its T-top for my drive home from the hospital. The cold Boston air was almost baptismal, allowing me to be cleansed daily of my own sometimes-thwarted efforts to clear the hospital roads of disease.

I never lost that almost physical need to be reborn at the end of the day. A few years after selling the Del Sol, I bought the car I always coveted in high school—a 1984 Porsche 911—on eBay, for a song. My family thought it was great. My in-laws, though, were aghast.

"How can you buy a car sight unseen, especially one from California?" my father-in-law demanded. He restored old cars as a hobby, and even paid for my wife's college education with the proceeds from a 1940 Ford he made look new again. After I proposed to my wife, he had me drive her around in his 1929 Ford Model A, a test of my worthiness. He neglected to tell me the car had a reverse shift. Meanwhile, the route he "suggested" for us required me to make the car come to a complete stop while ascending the steepest hill in rural Greensburg, Pennsylvania, and then to get it going again. I passed, though just barely.

"A lot of people buy cars online now," I told him. "I even had the seller take it to a garage, and the mechanic said it checked out fine."

"Hunh!" he scoffed. "The mechanic is probably in cahoots with the guy."

He and half the male population of Greensburg over the age of 70 were probably rooting against me, hoping that this car would be a lemon. But when it arrived it started right up, and never gave me a lick of trouble.

As my father-in-law's best friend of more than 60 years put it, "It must be feel great to be young and stupid."

Which passes for a compliment in those parts.

I got into the old Porsche and drove home, letting the Cleveland air work its magic. It wasn't entirely successful, though. I felt guilty knowing I was tooling around in a convertible, while Joan and David wouldn't breathe fresh air for weeks to come.

The next morning I was paged on the way to work by Karl from pathology. Always tricky to dial a phone while working a car's stick shift, but Karl never paged just to chat about the latest research in the journal *Blood*. I called him back at the next red light.

"Hiya. Good news, I think this lady has APL," he told me.

"Ms. Walker? Really? You have the FISH results back?"

Pennina Langer-Safer, M. Levine, and David Ward first developed FISH, or fluorescence in-situ hybridization, at Yale University in the early 1980s. With this test, a probe is manufactured to precisely fit a particular genetic abnormality within the chromosomes. Imagine a key that can only fit one genetic lock. Because these abnormalities are too small to be seen with the naked eye, even under a microscope, the probe is attached to a fluorescent marker that can be detected through the scope's viewfinder. The good news about FISH is that it is so precise, it can detect one cell out of a thousand with that genetic abnormality. The bad news is that it can only detect the one abnormality for which it was constructed, and will not detect other genetic mutations.

"Not yet. We should have that this afternoon. But these promyelocytes are classic. I noticed her coags are off, too, and she's got some schistocytes in her smear." Schistocytes are red blood cells that look as if someone used shears to make the ends of the cell jagged. Karl, gentle as usual, was telling me she had DIC without making me feel bad, in case I had missed it.

"Nothing gets by you, Karl. Somebody paged me about that last night, and we've already given her some cryoprecipitate." I replied, mentioning blood products that help restore the body's clotting factors, which are consumed as part of DIC. "You sure enough about this diagnosis for us to start her on some ATRA?"

"I think that would be a good idea," he answered. "We'll know more later today."

By this point I had reached the hospital. I parked, walked to my closet to exchange my outerwear for my white coat, and headed to the leukemia floor through my habitrail. Rachel was sitting at the nurse's station by a computer.

"Did the lab call you?" she asked.

I nodded. "Looks like this may be your first patient with APL."

"Awesome. Can you cosign the ATRA I ordered in the computer?" She never missed a beat.

I grabbed one of the WOWs, checked the dosing and schedule (twice a day, half the total dose in the morning, half in the evening, every day until she entered a remission, hopefully), and completed the order. "Let's tell her the good news before the pills arrive."

Joan was sitting in a chair by the door, reading *The Plain Dealer*. She glanced up at us as we walked in.

"Uh oh, it's never a good sign when the two of you walk in," she said, grimly. A spent bag of cryoprecipitate was still hanging on her IV pole, along with a bag of saline, and some zosyn, an antibiotic. She had spiked a fever, and not knowing whether it was due to the leukemia or to a brewing infection, we always played it safe and treated it as if it were infection. A couple of plastic caps from the ports on the IV lines were still lying on the floor. It had been a busy night for her. Behind her bed, a collection of menacing-looking connectors stuck out from the wall, labeled *air*, *oxygen*, and *suction*. Precautions? Or a herald of events not yet realized?

I smiled. "You know, we're not always harbingers of doom. Sometimes we bring good news."

A look of hope flashed across her face. "You mean I don't have leukemia?"

I could have kicked myself for being sloppy with my language. Good news is relative: this sure as hell wasn't good news compared to not having cancer.

"I'm sorry, you do have leukemia, that hasn't changed. But it looks like you have the relatively good kind of leukemia, the APL we talked about last night. We'll be 100 percent sure this afternoon."

She processed what I said for a few seconds. "Of course, I knew I had those blasts and the high white blood count. How could I have been so dumb?"

I shook my head. "Not dumb, Joan, nobody would ever call you that. It's just a lot of information, even for one of us to keep track of."

She nodded and exhaled, giving herself permission to be human for the moment. "Okay, next steps?"

I told her about the ATRA and the FISH test. "And then we'll start chemotherapy today, like we discussed."

"Would you consider treating her with arsenic?" Rachel asked. Joan looked at her in horror, and then at me, as if wondering what had prompted me to invite this she-devil into her room.

But, as usual, Rachel had been doing her reading.

Arsenic compounds have been used medicinally in Eastern and Western medicine for almost 2,500 years. Hippocrates treated ulcers with the yellow sulfide of arsenic, also called orpiment or realgar. In traditional Chinese medicine, arsenous acid or arsenic trioxide paste was often applied to treat "tooth marrow disease." Arsenic has been a treatment for the plague and malaria, and was used by Thomas Fowler at the end of the eighteenth century, in the form of potassium arsenite, to treat a variety of conditions, including rheumatism, epilepsy, hysteria, dropsy, heart palpitations, syphilis, ulcers, and cancer. In the nineteenth and early twentieth century, it was the standard therapy for syphilis, until it was replaced by penicillin. Well into the twentieth century, arsenic was even used to treat CML and Hodgkin lymphoma, after it was demonstrated in Boston in the 1880s that it could reduce high white blood cell counts.[5]

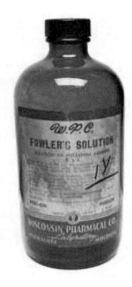

Figure 4.2
Fowler's solution, or potassium arsenite, used to treat a variety of health ailments from 1786 to 1936.

The empirical use of arsenic as an anti-leukemic agent continued in China during the past century. Then, in the late 1990s, Chinese investigators at the Harbin Medical University reported striking results when they treated APL patients with arsenic, absent additional chemotherapy: 73 percent of patients entered a remission, and even 50 percent of APL patients whose cancer had relapsed achieved this hallowed state. Around the same time, doctors in Shanghai reported similar results in patients whose APL had relapsed. Like ATRA, arsenic helps the leukemia cells stuck in primary school to mature and develop into high schoolers—healthy white blood cells. This led to a study in 40 patients treated with arsenic in the United States, all of whom had relapsed APL. Remarkably, 85 percent achieved normalization of blood counts and 86 percent even had disappearance of the translocation of chromosomes 15 and 17.[6]

As if the leukemia had never been there to start with.

Other studies were conducted in, of all places, resource-strapped India and Iran, where patients with a new diagnosis of life-threatening acute leukemia often had to wait days, at home, because no hospital bed was available for them.[7] Medical arsenic, though, is cheap, and can be administered outside of the hospital, because it has few side effects—other than its name. Remissions were achieved in over 85 percent of patients, 65 percent of whom were still alive five years after their diagnosis. Patients in these countries who previously would have died from their leukemia instead were cured thanks to this old, scary-sounding drug.

Arsenic was approved in the year 2000 for the treatment of relapsed APL in the United States, based only on that 40-patient study, because the results were so remarkable.[8] As occurs commonly with the introduction of new cancer drugs, studies start in patients who basically have no other options, and are the most desperate for a new therapy, and then are conducted in newly diagnosed patients, hopefully to prevent the cancer from ever recurring in the first place.

In the United States a nationwide study of almost 500 patients randomized them to receive arsenic, or not, following the initial round of aggressive inpatient chemotherapy (the cytarabine and daunorubicin). The investigators on that study found that patients who received the arsenic after they had achieved a remission from the chemotherapy were 20 percent more likely to be alive without the leukemia returning three years after their diagnosis than those who had not received the arsenic.[9] This was the treatment approach we were proposing to Joan Walker.

Meanwhile, in an even bolder study, investigators led by Elihu Estey, MD, at the MD Anderson Cancer Center were eliminating the use of traditional chemotherapy altogether, treating lower-risk APL patients (frequently defined as those who had low white blood cell counts and relatively higher platelet counts) at diagnosis with just arsenic and ATRA. Of the 25 patients they treated, 24 achieved a remission.

Without a drop of chemotherapy.

German and Italian investigators, under the lead of Uwe Platzbecker, MD, and Francesco Lo-Coco, MD, picked up on this finding and conducted a study of 156 patients with lower-risk APL who were randomized to receive a regimen similar to what Estey had pioneered versus standard chemotherapy. They presented their findings at a plenary session of the American Society of Hematology in 2012 in Atlanta, Georgia, in front of almost 20,000 hematologists.[10]

The results? Not only was the combination of ATRA and arsenic at least as effective as standard chemotherapy; it was more effective, and caused patients to actually live longer than those treated with chemotherapy. All 77 patients receiving the arsenic and ATRA went into a remission, compared to 95 percent of those receiving chemotherapy. At two years following diagnosis, 99 percent of patients treated with the arsenic and ATRA were still alive, compared to 91 percent for those receiving chemotherapy.

When Platzbecker showed the results, first of the similar remission rates, and then a graph with the line indicating survival for those treated with just arsenic and ATRA hovering over the survival line for those treated with chemotherapy, an audible gasp went up in the audience, as those of us attending realized that our standard treatment for people with lower-risk APL had just changed.

Fittingly, when their publication of the study results appeared in the *New England Journal of Medicine*, Zhu Chen, who had done so much to make ATRA the standard therapy for APL, wrote the accompanying editorial.[11]

So, why not use arsenic along with the ATRA to treat Joan Walker? I explained some of this background information to Joan.

"Unfortunately, your white blood cell count was really high when it was measured down in Wooster, and your platelet count was low. Our labs have shown the same. You have what we would consider to be a higher-risk version of the leukemia, and just giving arsenic and ATRA may not be enough. We'll need to give the chemotherapy along with the ATRA, and then, once you're in remission, we'll start the arsenic, as an outpatient." Just like in the nationwide US study.

"My luck, having the high-risk good leukemia." Joan shook her head, a gesture of incredulity. "Well, at least I have my health," she said, wryly. We all sat in silence for a bit, as

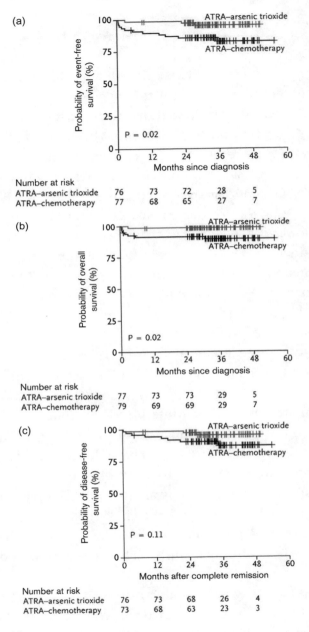

Figure 4.3
Improved survival for patients with acute promyelocytic leukemia treated with arsenic and all-*trans* retinoic acid (upper line) compared to patients treated with chemotherapy (bottom line). (a) Better event-free survival

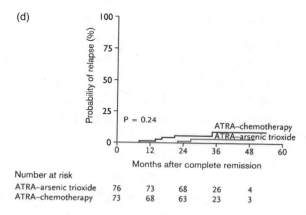

Figure 4.3 (continued)
(fewer events of death or leukemia relapse). (b) Better overall survival. (c) Better disease-free survival (less leukemia relapse). (d) Fewer leukemia relapses.

she continued to process what we had just discussed. "You did say remission, and that I would make it home."

"That's the goal. More likely than not, you'll get there."

"Promise?" she asked. Her eyes were both beseeching and commanding. Part patient, part OR nurse.

I hesitated, wanting to reassure her but also trying to be careful not to make absolute guarantees. "I promise we will do everything we can to get you through the chemo and then get you home."

She continued to stare at me, making clear that what I had said wasn't enough. I took a deep breath before continuing. "I promise we'll get you into a remission and back home safely." She nodded, sank back into her chair, and thanked us for seeing her.

Our conversation nagged at me, though.

I have been pushed by patients in the past to make promises—promises that they wouldn't die in the hospital; promises that they would live long enough to see a grandchild born; promises of cure.

To become a doctor, I had to take about a gazillion standardized tests, in undergraduate and medical school, aptitude tests to get into those schools, three steps of medical boards tests, and two steps of specialty boards. As any grizzled test taker will tell you, when an answer to a multiple-choice question contains the word "always" (as in, "APL is *always* treated with chemotherapy"), that answer is invariably wrong.

Promises of a guaranteed medical outcome are a form of "always." Add to this accumulating years of having seen the unexpected occur in patients, and it's no wonder doctors and nurses are reticent to make promises we aren't sure we can keep to our patients.[12]

On the other hand, I recalled a patient I met early in my career whose voice filled my small exam room with confidence and optimism. He was a large man, well over six-feet tall, and had been a scion in the business world, used to being in charge. After we discussed his leukemia diagnosis and treatment options, he put one of his large hands on my shoulder.

"Doc, I want to hear from you that you're going to cure this thing and get me back to my family where I belong.

At the time I was taken aback, and tried to adjust his expectations, interjecting a series of caveats in an even, measured voice. He interrupted me.

"You're not gettin' it. I only want someone to treat me who is going to be fighting like hell, just like I am, and isn't going to stop until this cancer is licked. I'm not hearing that from you."

But I didn't want to be the kind of doctor people talk about: not the one who tells people they are going to be alive in five years, yet they die two months later; and not the opposite—the one who tells people to get their affairs in order (right now!) only to be mocked when they breeze into his clinic two (or more) years later.

People want their doctors to be honest, but many also look for hope and confidence from them. I have tried to walk that line: between unabashed support for my patients, emanating from the compassionate part of me that aches to alleviate their fears; to reality checks about the grim statistics of the chances of curing their leukemias. Otherwise, how could they trust me to always tell them the truth?

But I haven't always been successful.

Rachel and I joined the rest of the team, who were organized in an approximate scrum around the WOWs. We frequently debated what to call the lot of us. A pride, as with lions? Seemed over-confident, as did a shrewdness of apes. A murder, as with crows? Too ominous. Maybe we were like a flamboyance of flamingos. I looked over to the latest pair of post-call residents, who weren't exactly looking flamboyant as they leaned against their WOWs to keep from toppling over. A gaggle—that felt right.

"How's Mr. Sweeney doing?" I asked.

John, looking spiffy in a clean shirt and tie, had admitted David, and thus would follow him for the duration of his hospital stay or until John's rotation ended—whichever came first. Frequently, our patients outlasted our residents.

"He had a pretty good night. Some nausea to the chemo, though, and his hemoglobin dipped to 7.8, so we're giving him a transfusion today."

"Did he throw up?" When John nodded I asked, "You gave him something extra for the nausea?"

"Compazine," John answered. Embarrassing as it may be to admit, some say our greatest advances in treating leukemia over the past couple of decades haven't been new chemotherapy drugs, but rather better nausea medication so patients better tolerate the chemotherapy we have; and better antibiotics, particularly antifungal medications, which reduce the number of people who die while their blood counts are low from life-threatening infections.

"Let's go see him," I said, as the gaggle of our team entered his room.

David was lying in bed, propped up on one elbow with his head swaying over a barf bucket. He looked miserable. Betty hadn't arrived yet.

"I guess it would be foolish of me to ask how it's going," I said, as he glanced at us sideways. He gave us a half-hearted thumbs-up sign, the way football quarterbacks who've suffered a concussion signal the fans as they're being carted off the field.

"We're going to take care of the nausea," I told him. I glanced up at his IV pole and saw the bag of red blood cells hanging. "We're also giving you some blood, which I think will give you a little more energy."

He nodded slightly, limiting his movements so he wouldn't start retching again. "Just knock me out for the rest of it," he whispered.

"I wish I could. You'll sleep from the medications. I'm sorry about all of this, we'll try to make it better."

He nodded at us slightly again and closed his eyes as his nurse brought in a syringe filled with Compazine, and injected it into his IV line. We left quietly.

I worried about his becoming nauseated so soon after getting chemotherapy. Though I'd seen it happen before, and obviously it is a common side effect to the types of drugs we use to treat the leukemia, it was a bit unusual. Nausea can be complicated. Sometimes, when it's like the "upset stomach" kind of nausea people get from eating food that doesn't agree with them, it's because the chemotherapy causes gastritis, an inflammation in the stomach. Other times it may be "the room is spinning" kind of nausea, like the feeling people get when they lie down in bed and close their eyes after a night of heavy drinking or following a particularly chaotic ride at the Cedar Point amusement park. In that case the chemotherapy affects their sense of balance, which the brain and nervous system control.

Nausea that is psychological comes in a couple of flavors. The first is anticipatory nausea, which patients may experience prior to receiving chemotherapy that has caused them to be nauseated in the past, or when encountering something they associate with nausea-inducing chemo. I heard about one patient who was successfully treated for Hodgkin lymphoma, which requires a chemotherapy regimen given every two weeks for four months. Every time she came to the cancer center, she threw up soon after receiving the chemo. Before long, she started throwing up in the car as soon as she saw the cancer center building, just anticipating how the chemo she was about to receive would make her sick.

Years later, after she was cured, this same woman was in the airport and happened to run into the oncologist who treated her. When the oncologist went over to greet her, she immediately threw up on his shirt, perhaps successfully fulfilling the wishes of many a cancer patient! The association hadn't been extinguished, even years later.

Similarly, patients whose sense of smell is heightened due to chemotherapy have told me they can't stand the "fragrance" of the antibacterial soap we use in our hospital. They associate it with their pre-chemo exam, performed of course with my freshly washed hands.

The other type of psychological nausea my patients have experienced relates to the five stages of grief described by Elizabeth Kübler-Ross in her landmark book *On Death and Dying*.[13] People facing death—or as in the case of leukemia, any serious illness that represents the loss of health—progress on their way to accepting this new reality through a series of reactions that can occur in any order. These include sadness or depression, anger, bargaining, denial, and finally acceptance. Some people may not experience all or any of these stages. But because time is so truncated—from the point when a person first seeks medical attention for what seems like the flu, to the start of chemotherapy for leukemia—we often see patients march through at least some of these stages during their hospitalization.

Sadness may be obvious, especially in people who are tearful, and thus we keep a box of tissues close at hand at all times. But it may be subtler in those who withdraw from family and friends, or don't engage in medical decision-making. Anger can be challenging: some patients will direct it toward themselves, as if they somehow could have prevented the leukemia from arising ("I should have gone to the doctor earlier!"); others will turn it toward their family, which causes predictable matrimonial discord or estrangement ("I told you to bring in my Cleveland Indians shirt, not my Cleveland Brown's shirt!"); and others still toward current or past health care providers ("The food here stinks!" or "Why didn't my primary care doctor find the leukemia at my appointment months ago?").

Bargaining can be clear-cut ("God, if you help me get into remission, I will be a better Christian"). Or it may involve negotiation over tests or procedures ("I really don't want to go for a CT scan today. How about we schedule one for tomorrow instead?"). Denial takes a number of forms, from doubting the diagnosis ("Can you repeat the bone marrow biopsy to make sure?") to intractable nausea that can't be relieved with medications—a subconscious, visceral reaction to the cancer diagnosis that a person may not be outwardly acknowledging but is nonetheless attempting to rid himself of. Depression can manifest itself in similar ways.

One of my patients, a woman in her late 20s with the same APL as Joan, was nauseated every day for the entire month she was hospitalized, and even after she was discharged to her home. We tried every nausea medication we had and engaged some of our specialists in palliative care to help; gastroenterologists then used a scope to see if there was a mechanical reason behind her nausea, but to no avail. Multiple times during that hospitalization, she asked us to repeat her bone marrow biopsy to confirm she had leukemia, even after we showed her print-outs of the biopsy reports that clearly stated: *FINAL DIAGNOSIS: ACUTE PROMYELOCYTIC LEUKEMIA.*

We eventually had to readmit her to the hospital because she couldn't keep food down. Her mother, who cared for my patient's 2-year-old daughter during her initial hospitalization, brought the girl in to visit during this second hospital admission. Perhaps it was her return to the hospital and the memories from her first stay. Maybe it was seeing her daughter run around that hospital room, and realizing just how much time she had just spent without her. But suddenly she burst into tears and sobbed unabated for the next hour. We witnessed in real time her psychological breakthrough as she progressed from denial of her leukemia diagnosis to acceptance. That night she ate everything on her hospital tray, and never had a twinge of nausea for the remainder of her therapy.

I remembered what Rachel had said about David: "It's not right. He doesn't want to be here. He doesn't want to get the Ara-C and daunorubicin. He only agreed to it because his kids wanted him to be aggressive." She was right. And with the nausea and vomiting, his body may have been agreeing with her assessment and revealing his true wishes about treatment.

We continued rounding for the next three hours, and then stopped in to see Joan as a team. Enough time had passed that her chemotherapy was already hanging from an IV pole when we entered her room. She was sitting in a chair, staring out the window, and barely turned around when we came in.

"How's it going?" I asked as I snuck around her bed to try to make eye contact. She glanced over to me.

"It's going."

"Anything we can do for you?" I persisted.

She shook her head and turned back toward the window. Sadness.

Our final patient of the day was a 72-year-old man who had received the same chemotherapy regimen that David Sweeney was just starting. We tell people at the beginning of their hospitalization, as they are considering their treatment options, that with the 7+3, they can expect to spend between four and six weeks in the hospital, and he was coming hard on six. His blood counts showed no sign of recovery, and his bone marrow was a wasteland of emptiness.

We walked into his room, where his wife sat in a chair by his bed. Amazing how frequently this same picture is repeated in room after room. She gave us a half smirk as we glanced over to her husband, who lay in bed with the sheets pulled completely over his head and tucked underneath it, a life-sized, starched cocoon.

"Oh, that's normal for him," she told us. "On the ship, he had to sleep on a couch that was located directly under a vent. It was the only way he could keep warm."[14]

The cocoon shifted as he heard us talking, and a hand emerged to pull down the sheet. He smiled sleepily at all of the eyes staring down at him, recognizing how silly he must have looked.

He was captain of a barge that hauled iron ore for the steel mills across the Great Lakes, at a time when steel mills were still open. (This is how the Steinbrenner family made enough money to buy the New York Yankees, when their attempts to buy the Cleveland Indians in 1972 were foiled.[15]) He steered these massive vessels from the back ("aft," he liked to remind us landlubbers), staring out across a deck the equivalent of two baseball fields long.

"He'd be gone from March through October. I was one of the Lake widows!" She started to chortle but stopped herself, realizing how the leukemia could make that moniker all too real.

"That's a long time to go without seeing each other," I commented. "How did you get through it?"

"I missed her, but we'd meet up every month or two," my patient said, sitting up in bed to join the conversation. "She would track the ship's location." I looked over to his wife for confirmation.

"I knew what day they would set out from Duluth, and approximately when they'd be getting into Chicago," she said. "I'd pile the kids into the car and we'd go see him."

"For how long?" I asked.

"A day, maybe longer if the ship had some maintenance issues," my patient answered. "After the kids were out of the house, she'd join me for a week or two on the ship. That was better."

His wife nodded but said nothing. A picture hung on the wall, of the sun rising over one of the Great Lakes. I imagined that was often the scene he woke to on his ship. We all stared at it for a few moments, before my patient sighed and asked if his blood counts had improved.

"Nope, not yet," I answered. "Any day now."

"It's okay, we're not in a hurry," said this man used to waiting, used to the familiarity of one day looking much like the day before. Acceptance.

David's nausea persisted, stubbornly, for the rest of his week of chemotherapy, while Joan's sadness started to lift as more of her friends and colleagues streamed in. They were a funny bunch—aware of her impending alopecia, a group of nurses from the Wooster hospital had donned masks that made them look totally bald or like old men with grotesquely receding hairlines. Later, when Joan did lose her hair, a few actually shaved their heads in solidarity.

Joan's children came to visit after school, often brought by friends or by the family they were now staying with. Joan did her best to show them she was the same mom as she had been two weeks earlier, before her diagnosis, teasing them and asking the same questions about the mundaneness of their daily lives as she would have over the dinner table. But despite their tough exteriors—her son's tattoos on his arms and trucker's cap, and her daughter's multiple piercings— they looked scared, fragile even, like kids whose main source of stability was now broken.

On rounds a few mornings later, it was John's turn to discuss Joan. He frowned a bit before starting.

"She had a rough night. She became short of breath, so we had to put her on oxygen. She also spiked a fever."

"Did you get a chest X-ray?" Rachel asked.

John nodded. "It showed some patchy infiltrates, consistent with fluid overload from heart failure." He turned his WOW computer screen toward me. Fluffy clouds floated over the gray background of her lungs. "So we diuresed her to take the fluid off and added vancomycin [an antibiotic] to her meds. But her oxygen requirements increased by morning, so we switched her from nasal canulae to a face mask. She's now on 10 liters of O2."

"Yikes," I said. "Not good. How are her blood counts?"

He crinkled his nose. "That's the weird thing. Her white blood cell count had been going down from the chemotherapy, but it suddenly spiked up today."

I nodded. "Let's start her on decadron 10 mg twice daily."

John looked at me quizzically. "You thinking a COPD flare? I don't think she's a smoker." Chronic obstructive pulmonary disease is often the end result of the havoc smoking wreaks on lung tissue. Sudden exacerbations are treated with steroids like decadron.

I shook my head. "Nope. And I'm not thinking heart failure either in someone this young without a history of heart disease." I glanced over at Rachel, as a dawn of recognition spread across her face.

"This is differentiation syndrome, isn't it?" she asked. I nodded. "She needs to be on steroids!"

"Wish I had thought of that," I razzed her. "Let's go check on Ms. Walker."

When we walked into Joan's room, I noticed a new photo now hanging on her wall, printed from someone's computer; she was standing among her friends in her hospital room, laughing, the day they were all dressed in their bald wigs. Another photo, in a frame on her window seat, must have been taken a year or two ago; she was with her two children, all dressed up, at what looked like a wedding reception. A third photo by the window was a few years old: Joan with her surgical team.

I've long made it a habit to scan the walls of my patients' rooms, to try to gain some insight into what their lives are like outside of the sterile confines of the hospital walls.[16]

Most are pasted with photos of family and friends, like Joan's: significant events, like anniversaries or weddings; posed holiday photos, with matching outfits and frozen smiles; and my favorites, the casual or even goofy shots of my patients with full heads of hair, taken during a summer trip to the shore with their families, for instance, in which everyone looks tan and relaxed, or at a Halloween party, their smiles exaggerated to match their outfits.

I've cared for members of high school football teams or their coaches, whose walls are often adorned with large posters signed by all the players, or with photos of the team holding up signs saying "Kick leukemia's butt!" When one high school football coach was being treated for leukemia, his family, friends, and team organized a fundraiser in which they sold rubber bracelets with his name on it; that year I saw Urban Meyer (who at the time was coaching at the University of Florida) wearing one at their national championship game.

Religion is a common theme, and patients often display crosses or St. Christopher's medals in their rooms. Some turn to the religion of Marvel and DC Comics, pasting stickers of Batman, Ironman, Thor, Spiderman, and even the Teenage Mutant Ninja Turtle, Michelangelo, on their doors. I've seen them sporting Superman T-shirts, too—especially fitting given the Man of Steel's "true" birth in 1933 at the hands of Jerry Siegel and Joe Shuster, two teenage boys from Cleveland's East Side.

But most touching are pictures drawn by children or grandchildren, with bright yellow suns, electric green grasses, and rudimentary people, one always taller than the other. If I look closely, I notice the extra care given to drawing the smile, one as wide as can fit into the oval of the head—as if, with that smile, the child is willing a return to happiness, to how things were before the leukemia.

The love I see on the walls of those rooms is breathtaking, and a constant reminder of what my patients are trying to recapture. For those whose walls remain unadorned for the length of their hospital stay, though, I worry about the care they will receive when they are finally discharged from the hospital. We spend extra time with them when they leave, ensuring they will be safe.

Joan, lying in her hospital bed, looked quite different from the Joan in her photos.

She was laboring to breathe, with respirations at a rate of 30 or 40 per minute. I could see the muscles and tendons on her neck strain with the effort. Her face mask, attached to one of the projections marked "oxygen" coming out of the wall over her bed, was foggy with her breathing. She looked worse than I imagined.

"Joan," I said, sitting on her bed and leaning in close to her face, so she could hear me over the flow of oxygen. "The chemotherapy we're giving you, the ATRA, is working. It's making the leukemia cells mature to normal white blood cells. But there's a side effect. You have fluid in your lungs and you're spiking fevers. It's called differentiation syndrome."

I looked her in the eyes but couldn't tell if she understood me. All I saw was alarm, the kind that people display when they're not getting enough oxygen and feel like they're about to suffocate.

"Joan, you have fluid in your lungs from the ATRA. Do you understand me?"

She closed her eyes and nodded.

"We need to send you to the ICU so we can give you more oxygen, so you can make it through this." As soon as I said this, out of the corner of my eye, I saw John and Rachel leave the room quickly.

Her eyes sprang open—more alarm. She shook her head. The ICU was her greatest fear.

"Joan, I think this is just temporary. We're giving you steroids, and that'll make it better, but it may take a couple of days for the steroids to kick in."

She closed her eyes again and mouthed something to me, but I couldn't hear it. I leaned in closer, lifted her face mask slightly, and asked her to repeat herself.

"Promise," she whispered, between breaths. "You promised, go home."

I lifted my face away. Her eyes were wide open.

"We'll get you home." I reassured her, but not confidently.

She held my gaze for a second, as if assessing my truthfulness, and shut her eyes again as the ICU staff entered her room. They rolled in a red "crash cart" that contained breathing tubes of various sizes, a defibrillator machine with paddles, IV lines and solutions, needles and catheters, cardiac medications, and all the ancillary equipment they might need to resuscitate a person in extremis. About 8 or 10 people accompanied the cart, swiftly doing what needed to be done. A few of them moved the bedside table and chairs away from her bed, and someone unlocked the brakes on the bed's wheel to move it away from the wall so someone else could stand behind Joan, at the head of the bed, if it became necessary to place a breathing tube down her throat.

I hoped I was right.

Meanwhile, David was nearing the two-week mark since we had started his chemotherapy. His nausea had improved as he marched toward accepting his leukemia diagnosis, and the chemotherapy we had given to treat it. But also as a consequence of the chemotherapy his blood counts, low to start with, had taken a major hit. His total white blood cell count was now 0.3 (one-sixth of his baseline), his platelets were 8,000 (placing him at risk of spontaneous bleeding if we didn't give him transfusions every other day), and he had become dependent on red blood cell transfusions every few days.

I entered David's room and smiled at him and Betty as they sat side-by-side in chairs near the window. As usual, I glanced first at the photos and pictures decorating the sill. One was a shot of the family standing near a small grill in front of a tailgate setup: everyone wore Ohio State sweat-shirts; David and Eric held beers.

"I'm sorry you're going to miss the game this weekend," I said to them.

David shrugged. "It's okay. I told the kids to go and to text me updates. I tried to convince Betty to join them, too, and take a break from this place."

She had been by his side every day, entering the Leuke-mia Unit and walking past our team's gaggle each morning around 9, and heading back home after dinner. Like David, she seemed to have accepted his decision and dutifully recorded the details of our daily updates into her small notebook, in which she also wrote down questions from other family members. I couldn't imagine what it must have been like for her, during the lonely drive to the hospital when she prepared herself mentally for the day to come, or during the even lonelier trip back home. Sometimes, she stayed at the guesthouse near the hospital, where family members of patients, or patients themselves with frequent outpatient appointments, temporarily reside. Alone at night, I wondered, was she imagining that this might be practice for widowhood?

Whenever a patient of mine dies, I send a note to the family, many of whom I have gotten to know pretty well. I use the occasion to reflect on how my patient affected me, and how much admiration I have for the often-inspiring way he or she lived with this contemptible disease. I also reflect on how lucky my patient was to have such a supportive partner, when that is the case. It isn't always.

Occasionally, I'll get a letter or phone call in return, in which the partner asks to meet with me.

It's usually a wife, now a widow.

Often, the focus of these visits is the chance to ask "What if?"

"What if the cancer had been caught earlier?"

"What if he had chosen a different therapy?"

"What if the antibiotic had been started sooner?"

I never take these questions as an accusation of malpractice. Rather, they remind me of Joan Didion's heroic exploration in her 2005 book *The Year of Magical Thinking*, where she reviews the details of her husband John Gregory Dunne's cardiac arrest repeatedly, especially the report from the ambulance first responders.[17] Her questions, and those my deceased patients' partners, likely represent an iterative revisiting of events in the hope that doing so will change the inevitable outcome.

One of my patients, a minister, once observed that my role in people's lives was pastoral. In that spirit, I tried to reassure these women: they had been exceptional partners, helping their husbands make good decisions and supporting them unfailingly, and they could not have altered fate.

I once met with a widow and her two children, aged 10 and 13 at the time. Their dad had a terrifically aggressive form of leukemia, and had died around Christmastime.

"We want to get some closure," his wife told me. I asked the kids if they were okay coming to see me, or if they faced it with trepidation.

"We're okay," his daughter, the older of the two, answered. His son, a spitting image of my patient, was quiet.

I spoke to them as if I were talking to my own children, mentioning how much I liked their dad, and how I looked forward to seeing him and their mom. I told them what an awful disease he had, and how courageous he and all of them had been in facing it. I looked both kids in the eye and told them their dad talked about them all the time, and that he was so proud of them.

The son started weeping quietly, and wiped his eyes with the back of his hands. His mother rubbed his back gently.

"It's okay to be a little bit relieved that your dad has died," I reassured them. "Meaning that you don't have to worry about him being sick and hear about leukemia every night." The pastor in me tried to absolve. They nodded their understanding.

The four of us remained quiet for a bit. I noticed they were all tan and asked if they had gone on a trip recently.

My patient's widow told me that, when he was dying, her husband had urged his family to go to Florida, to their usual spring break vacation spot, whether or not he could join them. They had honored this wish. She then told me a story about how, on their first night there, they discovered a bottle with a cork in it by the water, washed up on shore, "As if he had sent it to us."

As a family, they wrote a letter to my patient, stuck it in the bottle and replaced the cork, and then my patient's son threw it in the water.

But it came back. As if my patient were returning the bottle to them and asking, "Are you sure you'll all be okay without me?" So his son threw the bottle in the water again.

"And this time it stayed," the son told me, his sight set somewhere in the distance, picturing the beach, the heft of the bottle, the space where it once was.

I realized, at that moment, how worried I had been about them, and how much I, too, needed to be absolved by them for not being able to help him more.

"My place is here," Betty said, smiling at me, and patting David's hand.

"We're doing this so I don't have to miss any games next season, right?" David asked, taking her hand in his.

I nodded and gave him my non-answer. "That's the goal." I was still shaken from making my promise to Joan. "Speaking of which, I believe you have a date with a large needle tomorrow."

Two weeks after starting an intensive chemotherapy regimen, we routinely perform another bone marrow biopsy to determine if the leukemia persists, because we can't always tell from the blood counts. If we see enough blasts in the bone marrow, we give more of the same chemotherapy, hoping that will do the trick. If all we see is a vast wasteland—a bone marrow with few cells remaining because of the nuclear bomb of chemotherapy we used to level the landscape—we wait for the bone marrow, and blood counts, to recover on their own. When we started down this path, I had quoted to David a chance of going into remission of around 50 percent. If we had to retreat him, the likelihood that we would be successful dropped.

David grimaced as Betty took out her notebook and read over what she had written on one of the pages. "Oh yes, my secretary here has reminded me of that fact," he said.

"Administrative assistant," she corrected him. "When will we get the results back from the biopsy?" she asked.

"As early as tomorrow afternoon, but if the pathologists have to perform some additional tests, a day or two after that." She recorded what I said.

"And then you'll start more chemo?"

"As soon as we hear that leukemia is still there. If it is," I added.

She wrote that down too.

The following morning, Rachel performed his bone marrow biopsy. Betty had come in early, so she could be there for him. I asked Rachel how it had gone.

"He asked me if we had a punch card, so that every time he underwent a bone marrow biopsy, he could get one free," she answered. We all laughed—the BOGO (buy one, get one) nobody wants.

But we weren't laughing that afternoon when my pager went off and Karl's number appeared. It usually meant that the blasts persisted if results came back early. I gave him a call.

"Bad news," he said. "Mr. Sweeney still has 20 percent blasts."

"No need for additional tests to make sure?" I asked, half-heartedly. At this high a percentage, Karl was sure.

"Afraid not," he answered.

I thanked Karl and hung up the phone. As I promised David, and every patient we treat, there would be no delay in letting him know the results, good, bad, or otherwise. I marched into his room, where he was lying in bed, wearing an "Old Guys Rule" T-shirt and reading on his iPad. Betty sat in her usual chair, completing a crossword puzzle.

"Hey," I said to them as I walked over to sit at the edge of his bed. Betty, ever his protector, had her antennae up for danger. She had divined, either from my facial expression or from the unusual time of my visit, that information was about to be conveyed—information that would affect David's course. She put the puzzle down and took out her notebook. We had started calling it "The Book of David."

"What's going on?" she asked, her pen poised for action.

"I got a call from pathology. Unfortunately, the leukemia hasn't gone away, and we're going to have to give you more chemotherapy to try to get rid of the few remaining cells," I told them.

"How many are left?" David asked. I conveyed what Karl had told me. Betty flipped through her notes.

"He started with 42 percent. So that's less than half."

I nodded my agreement. "You're spot-on. We've made some progress, but we need to get those blasts to less than 5 percent."

"It's good that his blasts have come down so much though, right?" Betty asked. "How does this affect his prognosis?" She persisted, looking quickly at David and then back to me.

My colleagues and I researched how this situation affected the prognosis in more than 1,500 people with AML who had been treated in studies conducted by one of the National Cancer Institute (NCI) cooperative groups—the Southwest Oncology Group.[18]

The concept of cooperative group trials came about in 1955, when the NCI formed a Clinical Studies Panel that concluded cancer research would progress faster if cancer centers worked together to enroll patients—particularly those with rare cancers—onto the same studies. Congress appropriated $5 million to the NCI to create the Chemotherapy National Service Center, which organized a number of these cooperative groups around the country. The trials that emerged from these groups set the standards for care for a variety of cancers and helped debunk the utility of particularly aggressive (and disfiguring) treatments such as radical mastectomy for breast cancer, or certain particularly aggressive chemotherapy regimens for lymphoma, which led to higher rates of infertility and secondary cancers—meaning, the lymphoma treatment led to the development of other cancers years later—but worked no better than standard regimens.[19]

A little more than one-third of the 1,500-plus AML patients were in the same tough spot as David—with more than 5 percent blasts two weeks into their treatment with cytarabine and daunorubicin. As it turns out, no single factor predicted the ability of someone with persistent leukemia to enter a remission subsequently—from the absolute percentage of blasts remaining in the bone marrow, to the percentage reduction in blasts from where they started, to a person's age. Also, having persistent leukemia at this time point did not always portend a worse prognosis, but it exposed a person to risks associated with receiving more chemotherapy.

I communicated all of this to Betty and David. David still didn't look pleased.

"So I'll have to spend even more time in the hospital," he said.

"I'm afraid so. We'll give you another two days of the daunorubicin and five days of the cytarabine, and it'll take longer for your blood counts to recover as a result. Figure at least an extra week, maybe more."

David stared out the window, at the world he had left behind to receive this treatment that hadn't worked yet, the world he wanted to return to. Had he rolled the dice and lost? Or was it another test of his mettle, of what he was willing to endure for his family?

Betty had stopped taking notes and crossed her hands over "The Book of David." Staring at him, worry clouded her face. Would these be the last days together when they could still cling to a modicum of hope that the treatment would work? Or would it be one of the darkest hours they would look back on ruefully, years from now, when they knew that it had?

5
The Power of Her Fragility

nothing which we are to perceive in this world equals
the power of your intense fragility: whose texture
compels me with the colour of its countries,
rendering death and forever with each breathing

—e e cummings,
"somewhere i have never traveled, gladly beyond," 1959

"I'm warning you Anthony, cool it!" A woman's voice.

"Listen to your mother, Anthony!" Deeper, a man's voice.

I paused, my hand raised to knock on the exam room door, on my way to see Ms. Badway in the new cancer building. A couple of weeks had passed since she was discharged from the hospital, and I had already heard from her outpatient nurse, Jackie, that she had filled her prescription for the imatinib and had been seen in the high-risk OB clinic for what would become her weekly visits there.

The dynamic in the exam room sounded like one that might have emanated from any of my own family's outings. I knocked and entered.

Ms. Badway was walking to the trashcan to throw out some paper towels. A boy who looked to be about 4 years old, presumably the now-famous Anthony, was sitting on a stool across the room wearing a green shirt with the Hulk on it. He clutched a juice box. A couple of empty gummy bear packages were strewn nearby.

"Sorry doc, cleaning up a spill," she said, shooting a look at the boy. "This is my son Anthony and Joe, my husband."

Joe looked to be in his late 30s and wore loose jeans with a wine and gold Cavalier's T-shirt that read "The Land." He gave me a broad smile and a bone-crushing handshake, and then also shot a look over at his son.

"Anthony, what are you doin'? Get out of the doctor's chair!"

It reminded me of the time my wife and I took my children to their doctor's appointment, when my older son was 8 years old. As we waited for the doctor, he bopped around the exam room, as I'm sure Anthony had just been doing, while we sat in the available chairs. He suddenly stopped and looked around.

"Where can I sit?" my son asked.

I motioned to the doctor's stool. "Why don't you sit there?"

"I can't," he said. "That's where the doctor sits."

"Well, what do you think happens when I walk into a room to see my patients and someone is sitting on the doctor's stool?"

His eyes widened as he imagined the catastrophic fallout from this extreme breakdown of the rules governing social etiquette in his father's exam room. "I don't know, what do you do?"

I shrugged my shoulders. "I sit somewhere else."

I made my way to hop up on the exam table and told Anthony he could stay where he was. He opted instead to jump into his mother's lap as she sat down in a chair near Joe.

"Anthony, Jesus, be careful of your mother's stomach!" Joe barked at him. The kid couldn't catch a break. I tried to imagine the stress they were under, with three children at home, one on the way, a bunch of new doctor's appointments now added to their schedule, and the first time walking into a building that had the words "Cancer Center" on it.

"How's it been going Ms. Badway?" I asked. She laughed.

"*Mrs. Badway* is Joe's mother. Call me Sarah." I make it a point to never call my patients by their first names unless invited, wanting to be respectful of those who prefer the formality of a professional relationship. Those are mostly my older patients, and some of them still came dressed to the nines for their doctor's appointment. But I don't make assumptions about my younger patients.

"Fine, good to be out of the hospital, though I miss the peace and quiet of that place," Sarah continued.

"You doing okay with the pills?"

"Yeah, thank God we have insurance!" she answered, as Joe whistled.

"Wow, 12,000 bucks a month those cost! We only had a copay of $50. But 12,000 bucks? What do people do if they don't have insurance?' Joe marveled.

We had checked to make sure her insurance would cover the pills before she left the hospital. The cost of Gleevec, the brand name for imatinib, has risen steadily since it first came on the market in the United States in 2001. At that time, it was priced at around $2,500 per month. And while $30,000 per year isn't cheap, it's almost understandable given the exigencies of the time: although there was no competition for this miracle drug that made it unnecessary for most patients with CML to have bone marrow transplantation (a procedure that, all in, could run $500,000), there was some need to recoup research and development costs—both for imatinib, and for similar drugs that never made it to market.

What happened subsequently to its pricing, however, is unconscionable.

As with other specialty drugs, the cost of Gleevec rose at an approximate rate of 15 percent per year, and then sky-rocketed to its current levels for the two years prior to the drug coming off patent, which occurred in 2015, and just afterward. This is a common practice among pharmaceutical companies, to squeeze every last ounce of profit from a drug before there is adequate competition from generic versions of the same drug. Another common practice is to stonewall the requests of generic drug companies to obtain brand drug samples from which they can develop a generic version.[1]

Celgene, which manufactures the drug lenalidomide, or Revlimid, to treat multiple myeloma and myelodysplastic syndromes, has been lambasted for this practice—and for increasing the price of lenalidomide 145 percent over time.[2] Having to pay for the resources necessary to bring a drug to market might explain some pricing inflation at first, but that justification doesn't hold much water a decade after the fact. After all, when you buy a Ford Focus, even years after its introduction to the marketplace, are you also paying for every version of a Ford car that never reached a showroom floor?

One estimate places the number of people in the United States living with CML at 30,000. At the initial pricing of imatinib, the annual revenue from sales would have been almost $900 million—more than enough to recoup research and development costs within two years. Yet the price continued to climb.

It should come as no surprise that other drugs in the same class of tyrosine kinase inhibitors (the second- and third-generation TKIs that followed imatinib) have been priced comparably, rendering moot any decision-making based on economic efficiency for drugs with similar efficacy and toxicities. Unfortunately, generic competition has not impacted that pricing as much as was anticipated.[3]

Groups of hematologist-oncologists (myself included) have protested these types of wanton pricing of cancer drugs, with one scientific publication authored by more than 100 of us decrying the average escalation in cancer drug prices of $8,500 per year over the first 15 years of the millennium.[4] The drug cost for each additional year lived for

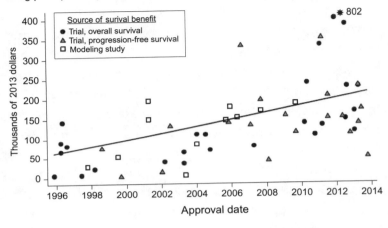

Drug price per life year gained versus drug approval date

Figure 5.1
The costs cancer patients must pay for drugs have risen dramatically since 1995. *Source*: figure 2 in D. E. Howard et al.; see note 3.

a cancer patient, which was $54,000 in 1995, skyrocketed to $207,000 in 2013.

In other words, 18 years later cancer patients are paying almost four times as much to live one year more than they would have without chemotherapy. And on average, 20 to 30 percent of that cost is paid out of pocket by those same cancer patients.[5]

Until there is federal legislation to rein in drug costs (as is done in parts of Europe, where pricing is part of the regulatory approval process), it is unlikely that the industry will respond to even a large group of well-meaning physicians unless there are cheaper alternatives that work just as well with a similar side effect profile. Pricing reform of cancer drugs will require changes from FDA and government regulators, in legislation, patent laws, reimbursement approaches, drug purchasing practices, and insurance and pharmaceutical companies.[6]

At the end of the day, we still need to treat our cancer patients, and continue to prescribe expensive drugs while we grind our teeth at the individual and societal cost of doing so.

"There are some patient assistance programs that help out," I told Joe. "And some patient organizations that will help with a limited amount of costs. Some folks even sign up for Medicaid to help cover their treatment."

"But there are also people who still can't afford their medicines," Sarah said. I nodded as she and Joe shook their heads, as if incredulous that people in this country and in this day and age still had to forgo cancer treatment.

"Any side effects to the pills that you notice?" I asked her.

"I get a little nauseous, like during my first trimester, but that's about it." I suggested she take the imatinib with the biggest meal of the day, which often helps with the nausea.

"Have you missed any pills?" I followed up.

Before coming into the exam room, I had noticed that her white blood cell count had decreased from 330,000 to 248,000, and that her platelet count had come down a bit, from 470,000 to 420,000—an improvement from where she started, but not as much as I usually see after a couple of weeks of imatinib. Anthony had started to get restless and was banging a matchbox car on the desk that held the computer. Sarah held his arm steady and he started to squirm: *Hulk strong.*

"Only a couple," she answered. Anthony slid down from her lap and was sitting on the floor. He seemed to be calculating his next move: *Hulk free.*

"How many is 'a couple'?" I persisted.

"A few," she said. That couldn't have left many days in the past week when she did take them. "But it's hard to remember, what, with everything else I have to do around the house."

"You haven't been taking your chemo?" Joe asked.

"Get off my back, Joe. How 'bout you do the laundry and I'll take the chemo?"

When all of those people with CML were enrolled in those large studies that led to imatinib's approval, in the years from 1998 to 2000, almost all had blood counts that returned to normal, and most had at least a reduction in the amount of Philadelphia chromosome that could be measured. Many even had complete elimination of the genetic abnormality.

Over time, some patients "lost their response"—their CML returned. A group of investigators from Belgium wondered what had happened, what could have caused this miracle drug to fail.[7] So they designed a study that included more than 200 CML patients treated at 34 centers, and administered adherence questionnaires to both the patients and their doctors. A pill count was then performed to confirm questionnaire responses. Approximately one-third of patients were non-adherent for the 30 days prior to the study and for the 90-day study duration. Interestingly, of those who were non-adherent, most (71 percent) took less of the drug than they should have, but almost 15 percent took more—either through an honest misunderstanding of how much to take, or because of a belief that taking more would work better to eliminate the leukemia. Of those with suboptimal responses to imatinib, 23 percent reported missing doses of the drug, compared to 7 percent of those with optimal responses. Patients whose CML returned were significantly more likely to have missed doses than those who maintained their response to imatinib. And the likelihood that the CML returned increased with the more pills that were missed.

Medication adherence is a problem in any chronic medical condition. One study of more than 30,000 patients taking statin medications for high cholesterol estimated that only 43 percent were taking their pills as directed after six months.[8] A study of almost 8,800 women taking hormonal therapies for breast cancer found that they were adherent only about 50 percent of the time.[9]

Another study conducted in the United Kingdom at Hammersmith Hospital provided 87 CML patients with pill bottles that contained their imatinib prescription, but didn't tell patients that the investigators had installed a microelectronic monitoring system—a computer chip—in the bottle's cap.[10] The chip recorded every time the patient unscrewed the bottle to remove an imatinib tablet, thus measuring their medication adherence.

The results? Medication adherence was better among these dedicated patients, at almost 98 percent. Those with adherence rates less than 90 percent, however, were significantly less likely to achieve a remission than those with better adherence rates. To put this in perspective, as imatinib is a once-a-day pill, a person would only have to miss four pills per month—one per week—to compromise the chance of entering a remission.

Not surprisingly, when people like Sarah have busy lives that get busier, they are more likely to forget to take their imatinib. At one presentation at a medical conference in Chicago one of the study authors, Dr. Jane Apperley, showed a slide of one man's adherence during December and January. As the frantic pace of the holidays approached, his pill taking fell off, and he missed multiple doses of imatinib. Then, starting January 2 (and probably as a result of a New Year's resolution), his adherence improved markedly, and he became a model patient.

I'm terrible at remembering to take pills, so to me this is completely understandable. I have other CML patients, though, to whom such behavior is incomprehensible.

"Miss a dose?" they have responded when I ask the same question of them that I did of Sarah. "It's cancer and this is my chemo. I would NEVER miss a dose!"

The problem—and it's a good problem to have—is that people with CML who take a drug like imatinib and who have restoration of their blood counts start to feel so good, like they don't have leukemia at all, that they forget that it's the pill that's making them feel so good, and then they start dropping doses. This is the same phenomenon that occurred among HIV-positive patients who started taking anti-retroviral medications, many of whom rose like Lazarus from the near dead.[11] This happens particularly when people are on the medication for months, or even years.

Others stop taking their medication because they don't like the daily reminder that they have cancer, and that this cancer could kill them if not for these pills. Call it denial, or the subconscious going rogue. Some people do have significant side effects and take matters into their own hands to avoid them.

And still others skip doses, or cut tablets in half, because they can't afford the pills or their insurance copay. At $50, Sarah's copay was not low enough to qualify as negligible, but it was not terribly high. Some patients have told me that their insurance companies disingenuously agreed to cover the $12,000 monthly cost of imatinib, as long as my patients agreed to the $8,000 monthly copay.

"It's really hard to remember to take these pills, and everyone forgets some," I reassured Sarah. Joe seemed to relax a bit. Anthony got up from the floor and started to roam around the room.

I explained the importance of sticking to her schedule, and methods she could put into place to help remind her to take her pills—setting a daily alarm on her phone, placing the pill bottle in a location she will see, even associating taking the pills with another daily activity, like brushing her teeth. Anthony threw his car against the wall. *Hulk smash.*

"Is it okay for her to keep the pregnancy with the chemo?" Joe asked.

I turned to Sarah. "Are you worried about birth defects? Is that maybe affecting how many of the pills you're taking?" I knew we had discussed this in the hospital and that she had said that her health had to come first. But people can have second thoughts.

She stared down at her hands, clasped over the bump of her belly. "Maybe a little."

"Sarah, you didn't tell me that," Joe said, almost tenderly.

It reminded me of a similar interaction I had with another patient who had CML, a man, in the same exam room.[12] I had prescribed imatinib for him, too, but for some reason he hadn't done as well as most on the drug. His blood counts never quite reached normal values, and his Philadelphia chromosome stubbornly persisted.

His wife became pregnant while he was taking imatinib, and she accompanied him to an appointment with me. When she told me she was pregnant, it was without joy, and she quickly added that she was considering getting an abortion. When I asked why, my patient jumped in.

"We're worried about birth defects."

I told them what I wound up repeating to Sarah and Joe. That a National Toxicology Program publication (from the National Institutes of Health) reported rates of major congenital malformation for women exposed to chemotherapy during their first trimester of pregnancy to be 14 percent, but only 3 percent for exposure during the second or third trimester.[13] I tried to put these data in context of how difficult it is to determine, sometimes, if chemotherapy caused specific birth defects, given the background rate of 3 percent birth defects in the general population, according to the Centers for Disease Control and Prevention. Data on birth defects from men exposed to chemotherapy at the time of conception are even harder to come by.

My patient exhaled, relieved that the risk of birth defects in their unplanned pregnancy was low, despite his having taken the imatinib.

"That's good news." He smiled and held his wife's hand. Her face remained troubled, though, with worry etching dark lines in her young forehead.

"But what happens if I have this baby and he's not here to be its father?" She stared at me, unblinking, as tears streamed down her face. My patient stared across the room at neither of us, considering the brutal honestly of her question.

I acknowledged the uncertainty of my patient's future, as we struggled to find a drug that would get him into a remission. I also recognized the burden it would place on her, to have a newborn and a sick husband. There was another aspect to this terrible situation, though, that I'm sure she was also considering.

"If the worst happens, you'll still have a part of him that will live on," I told her.

They sat silent, holding hands, considering a world with him as a doting father, and one without.

And so it often goes in my exam rooms, where cold truths, moments of elation and despair, and people's deepest worries are revealed, sometimes for the first time. Sterile, unadorned, and bare as they may be, these rooms are also safe havens where people feel they can be honest, with me and with each other, and where they can be heard.

"Okay, I'll take the pills," Sarah said, now resolved.

"Really?" Joe asked.

"Yeah, I'll do it. I'll really do it," Sarah reassured him. And me.

Anthony stooped to pick up his car, stood back up, and whacked his head on the corner of the counter. He started wailing. *Hulk done with doctor visit.*

Afterward, Rachel met me in the outpatient clinic and we walked to the hospital together, to see Joan.

"She's better," Rachel said as we headed over, smiling and nodding every so often at people we knew who were walking in the opposite direction, good Midwesterner that I had become. "Her FiO2 is 21 percent"—the same oxygen percentage as the air we breathe, so that's as low as the ventilator will go. The highest is 100 percent, which can't be sustained for too many days, as it can damage the lungs—"and they're going to extubate her today." Remove the breathing tube. "The steroids really worked."

"I'm glad the differentiation syndrome is resolving. Is she awake?" I asked.

"Oh yeah. Writing her questions on a pad of paper by her bed, making sure the ICU nurses know what they're doing." I smiled, remembering an old joke: What's the difference between a surgical/ICU nurse and a bulldog? Fingernail polish. She was tough.

"Have her kids been in to see her?"

Rachel nodded as we entered the stairwell to walk from the third to the sixth floor. I force myself (and, by default, the residents and fellows I work with) to take the stairs if the distance we have to travel is within three flights up or five flights down. Otherwise, I'd never get any exercise.

It was once suggested to me, by a female resident, that perhaps I should invoke this rule only after having to follow it myself wearing heels. A fair point, but I wonder if she's come around yet in her career to the proverbial advice, "Wear sensible shoes."

"They've been by every day. The ICU was a wake-up call." Rachel answered.

Family members, too, go through the Kübler-Ross stages after a cancer diagnosis. I'm glad her kids had come around.

Rachel flashed her badge by the reader outside the ICU and the doors swung open. The noise from the unit struck us like a brusque wind. It took me right back to my first day of internship, when I met the woman who would convince me to become an oncologist.

That day would turn into the longest one of my life.[14] I met my junior resident, Dave, the person who would share my call nights, at 7 a.m. in the ICU. When I walked through the automatic doors that first time, the noise level surprised me: a constant garble of voices coming from the central nurses' station which was made even more indecipherable by the constant humming of floor buffers used by environmental services workers nearby; above all that, alarms sounded from breathing machines or cardiac monitors every time a patient's oxygen saturation dipped, or someone's breathing didn't sync with the ventilator, or when someone else's heart beat too fast or too slow. I walked by the bloated, wrecked bodies of the patients, feeling like a bystander on a World War II movie set when, after the battle, the camera pans slowly over the fallen troops so the viewer can better absorb the horror of the carnage.

Before my internship at Massachusetts General, the largest hospital in New England, I had never before seen people this sick. I would later learn that patients cared for in other hospitals' ICUs often came directly to the regular patient floors at Mass. General, so you had to be remarkably sick to make it into the ICU there. (The same is true at Cleveland Clinic, which is almost twice the size.) The sobering effect of such concentrated illness gave me pause. I then headed toward the narrow conference room at the far end of the unit.

When Dave and I arrived, there were three other intern–junior resident pairs sitting or standing around a thick, honey-colored wood table that dominated the room, along with a third-year ("senior") resident, a pulmonary and critical care fellow, and a couple of Harvard medical students. Two white boards, with what looked like oxygen-saturation curves and respiratory-flow equations written in red marker, hung on the walls, and a manikin was propped up on a side table with a breathing tube stuck in its mouth. There were also a couple of guys sitting at the end of the table who looked rough—hair disheveled, two-day growth of beard, light-blue scrubs untucked beneath their dirty white coats.

They held heavily wrinkled paper lists of patients in front of them, clutching them like sacred scriptures. This much hadn't changed between my residency then and John's now. I realized they were post-call—they had just spent the night taking care of all of these horribly sick people. Dave and I would be sitting in their seats in 24 hours. Looking like them.

"You guys ready for sign-out?" the post-call duo asked the rest of us in the room.

"Let's do it. You've got other services to pick up," answered the senior resident, Ben, with a laugh. It was true—after finishing with us, this disheveled pair would leave to care for patients elsewhere in the hospital.

One of them smiled, his eyes tired. He seemed to be forcing himself to respond with confidence.

"Yes we do! But you know what? At least we won't be spending the next month in the Deathstar!" Wow, was that crass. This is what they called the ICU. I wondered if I would become as jaded.

I looked around the room at my co-interns. We laughed with the rest of the crowd, but much more nervously.

"In bed 2 is Mr. Yankowicz, a 58-year-old guy with obesity, and a 60-pack-year history of smoking." I remembered from medical school how to quantify the amount a person smokes in the course of his lifetime: multiply the number of cigarette packs he smokes per day by the number of years he has smoked. So, 60 pack-years could mean someone smoked one pack per day for 60 years, or two packs per day for

30 years. During my training, I would meet people whose pack-years number reached triple digits.

The post-call junior resident stopped for a second, looked up from the Holy Grail papers on which this information appeared, and continued. "He likes Marlboros—for anyone who's interested—and he's got diabetes. He came in yesterday because of severe groin and leg pain and on ultrasound and CT scan was found to have a dissecting aorta down the femoral artery. Surgery said it wasn't bad enough yet to operate so they're holding off, he needs his pedal pulses checked every hour. We have him on Lopressor, his BP is 102 over 56, heart rate 74 . . ."

Dave was writing down this information quickly on his own patient lists, and drawing small, open boxes next to the tasks we'd have to perform that day, so as not to forget what had to be done. Check pedal pulses—at the feet. Follow blood pressure to keep the systolic less than 110, to minimize the chance that Mr. Yankowicz would continue to dissect his arteries. Call the surgeons to see when they would be ready to take him to the OR. Once each task was completed, he'd fill in the box and move on to others.

"Mrs. Flannigan, 68-year-old woman with COPD, coronary artery disease, 70 pack-years of smoking, admitted with pneumonia, total white-out of her right lung, on triple antibiotics and 2 pressors, vent setting with an FiO2 of 60 percent and climbing, pressure support of 20, PEEP of 10 . . ."

Dave was writing furiously. I didn't understand most of what this guy had just said, but I would within my first week. On a chest X-ray, air and fat look black, whereas bone, some fluids, and infection look white. So a "white out" of her lung meant that on her X-ray, her right lung was entirely filled with either fluid or infection, which was why she required a ventilator. Her FiO2 was closing in on that maximum of 100 percent. Pressure support was how forcefully the machine was getting the oxygen into the lungs, and PEEP—positive end-expiratory pressure—had to do with keeping the airways open to get the oxygen. She was also on pressors—medications to keep the blood pressure up. Ben interrupted him.

"Has anyone called a family meeting? This sounds like it's getting pretty futile."

"Yeah, we tried that," the post-call junior resident said. "They're a full go."

Ben shook his head, clearly bothered by the news that the patient's family wanted "everything done" to keep her alive. "I'll call them together again to talk it over. Maybe I can convince them otherwise."

I soon learned that these types of momentous family discussions were a daily ritual in the ICU for one or another patient's loved ones. At a certain point, the docs and nurses caring for a patient would recognize that the person's chance of ever making it out of the unit alive had become vanishingly small, and it was time to withdraw care and let nature take its course. A family meeting would be called, the gravity of the situation discussed, and most of the time the family would agree, particularly if they recognized, along with the medical staff, how aggressive the intensive care had already been. The docs and nurses would then stop further interventions—even checks of blood pressure or heart rate—and reduce the amount of blood pressure or ventilator support they were providing, until a patient died, ideally with the family by the bedside.

But occasionally a family would not agree with this assessment and insist that everything still be done—even as the ventilator and blood-pressure support was maxed out, and patients started to require kidney dialysis. Unfortunately, such interactions could even get hostile. Some families lost faith in the medical staff for wanting to withdraw care, while medical staff became resentful that patients were being subjected to care with little potential to help but high likelihood of harm—a violation of the Hippocratic oath. Now I can see both sides of these situations, as families hope for a miracle, and in truth I have seen patients recover against all odds. But I have also seen patients, at the behest of their families, who undergo procedures I would never want to have myself if I were living my last days.

Back then—during my internship and the remainder of my residency—I was "young and stupid," to quote my father-in-law's buddy. I hadn't lived enough of life to appreciate its preciousness, to have sustained decades-long relationships with another person to understand the devastation of their loss, or to have seen enough of the *against all odds* cases, particularly among my leukemia patients, who survived their stays in intensive care units. Back then I was more likely to invoke futility.

Sign-out took 45 minutes, and then Dave and I, and the other intern-junior pairs, went off to round on our patients.

No point in mincing words: I was completely and utterly useless. I didn't know how to use the computers to look up lab results. I didn't know how to read the flow sheets at the patients' bedsides to document extremes and averages of blood pressure, heart rate, temperature, systolic arterial pressures, wedge pressures, or pulmonary arterial pressures. I didn't even know how to write an order yet, and thank God a nurse was nearby to tell me how to prescribe potassium—my first prescription as a legit doctor. At the very least, I was able to sign it without her assistance. I didn't know how to fight the tubes and wires draped over my patients' chests so I could listen to their hearts or lungs with my stethoscope. It was completely demoralizing. After an hour of this, I actually checked my own hospital badge to make sure "MD" really and truly followed my name. It was, though I assumed it stood for "Major Disappointment."

Next came rounds with the whole team, including the staff doc, a guy named Dr. Thompson. Staff docs at Mass. General were called "visits" because in the nineteenth century, if you were wealthy and living in Boston, doctors would visit you in your home and not the other way around. Only poor people actually came to a hospital. Thompson was kind. He was decisive. He stopped rounds to teach us about lung dynamics. He was brilliant. And I felt totally out of my league. I again looked sheepishly at my co-interns, and was grateful that they seemed to have the same deer-in-the-headlights look as me. We interns would grab the green charts from the rack and hand them over the juniors. They were the ones who presented the patients while we shifted our weight from one leg to the other during the four hours until rounds were done. This was in the pre-WOW days. So Dave did all the work of summarizing what had happened with our patients over the past 24 hours, all the work of writing notes, of making decisions about patients, and of planning our day. I held the green charts.

We spent 30 minutes after rounds that day doing the most urgent tasks on Dave's list—he now had small open boxes that went all the way down three pieces of paper—and then we broke for lunch in the conference room as we were taught, once again, by the indefatigable Dr. Thompson. We spent the rest of the afternoon placing invasive lines, ordering tests, calling for consults, and speaking to family members. Well, to be clear, Dave did all of that while I held the green charts. I did run a couple of errands for him and was thrilled when I could successfully locate an X-ray in the catacombs of the radiology department! Nowadays, of course, X-rays and medical records are all on computers, so I can't imagine what first-day interns in the intensive care unit actually do with their time.

Most of that day is a blur, though I did notice Ben in Mrs. Flannigan's room, standing by the window with his arms crossed as he was talking to what I assumed were her family members, who were sitting across the room. One older man stood by the patient's bedside, holding her hand and crying.

As night fell, we rounded out, during which the other intern-junior pairs told us about their patients. We heard about a couple of new admissions, another old guy with a lot of medical problems, and now with a pneumonia, who might need to be intubated, and a woman with metastatic ovarian cancer who was having trouble breathing and might also need to be intubated. Dave scribbled a lot more notes on the same pieces of paper that had been our bible for the day (now with most of the small boxes filled in). Then, the other residents took their leave, a scene straight out of that same World War II movie that started my day. We had now arrived at the part in which the company is forced to abandon two guys whose legs got shot up, and leave them with a certain amount of ammunition to fend off the advancing Germans. The departing troops always say goodbye and promise to come back to retrieve the guys the next morning—if the two survive the night, which everyone knows is highly unlikely.

So, instead of the 6 patients we cared for during the day, we were in charge of 20. I was hoping that disease recognizes the need for sleep, too, and we would have an easy night, but it was not to be. The overnight bag I packed, including replacement contact lenses, glasses, a set of scrubs, toothbrush and toothpaste, a comb, and a change of underwear, would remain unopened.

Dave and I rounded, just the two of us, on all the patients so we could get to know them, at least by sight. At about 8:45, Dave told me to go get us some dinner.

"Where?" I asked. The cafeteria closed at 7 p.m.

"Down at the cafeteria. They have a special meal at 9 for the interns and residents. One of us has to remain in the unit in case a patient crashes, so if you'd like *I* can go instead and *you* can stay here." He smiled, knowing the suggestion that I remain alone with 20 sick patients would terrify me to the point of near incontinence.

I walked out the doors to the ICU and realized it was the first time I had exited in 14 hours. I then took the elevator to the basement and looked down the hall toward the cafeteria entrance, which was blocked by a garage-door gate that was pulled down tight. A gaggle of people were standing in front of it, waiting—interns and residents in internal medicine, surgery, pediatrics, psychiatry, emergency medicine, and pathology. The pathologists were standing closest to the gate. I recognized some co-interns from our orientation, and we shared a couple of war stories from the day.

At precisely 9 p.m., a cafeteria worker came over to slide up the gate. As soon as it was three feet off the ground, the pathology residents bent down and scurried under, making a beeline for the desserts. Really? Were they that delicious? Soon everyone pressed in. I grabbed a tray to scope out the selections.

It took me a few nights on-call to figure out how best to game the nighttime food selections. The "special meal" for residents represented what was left over from the day's selections—obviously, the least popular meal choices. Dessert consisted mostly of fruit-flavored Jell-O, but occasionally a couple of chocolate puddings would remain, and that's what the pathology residents were gunning for. We joked that by the end of residency, having eaten all of that Jell-O, we probably had the strongest fingernails of any internists in the continental United States. The leftover entrée selection was always nondescript white fish or the vegetarian special. For vegetables, we were treated to waxy green beans or the occasional wilted lettuce with Thousand Island dressing. I loaded up the tray and headed back up to the unit, glancing over my shoulder wistfully at my co-interns, who had the luxury of remaining in the cafeteria and sharing a meal together. It took me a little longer than others to get to know all the members of my intern class, because the ICU would be so isolating that month.

Back upstairs, I set the tray on the conference room table and found Dave. Almost immediately, the disasters began. Mr. Yankowicz cried out from Room 2. We ran in.

"What's going on, buddy?" Dave asked, cool as a cucumber. My heart was in my throat.

"My leg! My goddamn leg!" He was holding his right thigh. Dave grabbed a Doppler machine, which has a probe that you place over someone's pulse so that you can actually hear the *whoosh, whoosh* of blood coursing through an artery, and placed it on Mr. Yankowicz's foot. We heard his pulse only faintly, even when Dave turned the Doppler's volume all the way up.

"We better call the surgeons," Dave said. "I think he's dissecting his artery even further, and he's no longer getting any blood to the lower part of his leg."

Dave paged them and a couple of minutes later two guys in scrubs came into the unit, grabbed the Doppler, and put it on Mr. Yankowicz's foot. We again heard the same faint pulse.

"We'll operate tomorrow. As long as he's getting some blood to that foot, he's okay," the older surgeon said. The younger one looked about as terrified as me, and I assumed his internship had started that same day, too. Twice more that night, Mr. Yankowicz would cry out, and we'd go through the same procedure with the Doppler, verifying he still had a pulse. Early the next morning, he was whisked away to the OR.

As we were leaving his room, one of the nurses, Janet, came over to us.

"The new admission in bed 10 . . ."

"What's his name?" Dave interrupted her. A lot of docs and nurses had gotten into the habit of referring to patients by their bed numbers. The point was really to avoid using their names in public and thus violating the privacy guaranteed to every patient under the Health Insurance Portability and Accountability Act (HIPAA), which was just being passed by Congress and signed into law by President Bill Clinton that year.[15] But Dave believed they had gone overboard and in the process dehumanized people even further. He insisted on hearing everyone's name—a practice I would follow throughout my career, as well. The nurse rolled her eyes.

"Mr. Wilson, 78. Married. He likes long walks on the beach, quiet nights by the fire, and occasionally he likes to cuddle with his sweetheart."

Dave laughed. "I got it, I got it. Is there anything else he likes? Maybe a breathing tube?"

"Precisely," Janet answered.

"Alrighty then. We're a full-service hospital. Let's give the man his money's worth."

We followed Janet into Room 10. An elderly man with a white, grizzled growth of beard was lying in bed with a face mask plastered over his mouth and nose. He was breathing quickly, maybe 40 times per minute. His eyes looked anxious, and his hands were grabbing the bed sheets, as if he were trying to brace himself while he breathed. Dave stared at the monitor over his bed, and I followed his gaze to see it registering an oxygen saturation of 78 percent and a heart rate in the 120s.

"Mr. Wilson!" Dave shouted at the man. "We're going to have to put a tube down your throat to help you breathe! You can't keep going like this without one! Is this something that you want us to do?"

Mr. Wilson locked eyes with Dave and nodded quickly. Janet had already rolled a cart into the room with plastic tubes and some metal instruments on its surface. Dave moved behind Mr. Wilson's bed and lowered the head of it until it was flat. This did not help Mr. Wilson's breathing, and he shut his eyes. Dave spoke calmly but with authority as he took the mask off Mr. Wilson and sprayed an anesthetic into his mouth. It smelled faintly of oranges.

"Can I have a Mack and a 7.5 French tube." The Mack, short for Mackinaw, was one of the metal instruments on the cart. Dave pulled on the Mack's lever and a light came on. He stuck the lever into Mr. Wilson's mouth, deep, the light helping him to see where he was going, to press down on Mr. Wilson's tongue while the nurse handed him a plastic breathing tube. Dave slid the tube over the lip of the lever, then even deeper, past the vocal cords, and removed the Mack. He took a syringe and injected air into a port that came off the tube—this would inflate a collar around the tube that would keep it anchored in Mr. Wilson's throat. He attached the end of the tube, sticking out of Mr. Wilson's mouth, to the large tubes leading to the ventilator. Finally, he took his stethoscope and listened to Mr. Wilson's lungs, and in the area of his stomach, to make sure he successfully placed the tube into Mr. Wilson's trachea, and not his esophagus. We would get an X-ray to confirm the placement soon after.

"Sounds like a winner to me!" Dave said, as he cleaned up the packaging from the tube and instruments, and we left the room. Within the next week, I would learn how to do this myself, and eventually would place more breathing tubes in patients than any other intern in my class. But at that moment, I just stood in the room with my mouth open. I think I had just witnessed Dave saving this guy's life.

"You ready for some grub?" Dave asked me. I looked at my watch. It was almost midnight. He went ahead to the conference room as I lagged behind, glancing into the rooms of these patients I was now officially helping to care for.

I stopped as I passed the room of Mrs. Abrams, the woman with ovarian cancer whose lungs were filling with fluid. She was a pediatrician from a nearby hospital. Initially, she was to be intubated and placed on a respirator, but she had changed her mind, deciding instead to live her last hours breathing air on her own, unassisted. She was in her early 40s, and her appearance in our unit had ruled our team's emotions that day. It didn't help matters when her son and daughter, ages 10 and 8, came in to say goodbye to her in the evening—we all knew this would be the last time they would see her. Each of us in turn, doctors and nurses, sought refuge off the main floor to check the hitch in our breathing or cry outright in private. I had never been witness to this kind of family drama up close, and it was heart wrenching.

Just before we had rounded out with the rest of the team, her husband escorted their children away and returned a couple of hours later with her best friend, now carrying a bag from CVS. As I was doing my rounds, checking vitals on patients to dutifully report back to Dave, I glanced in her room and saw her husband standing, hunched over her bed, holding a clipboard while she struggled to write something. I made it back to our conference room.

"Hey Dave, what's going on in there?" I asked, gesturing to her room. By this point in the day I had proven myself to be so utterly helpless that I no longer even worried about asking Dave completely idiotic questions. He was my life-line, my only source of truth. Even if I'd had time to use the bathroom, I probably would have needed his assistance there too. He looked at me blandly, but without prejudice.

"She's writing out cards."

"You mean 3×5 cards?" I asked. I had a pocket full of them, each with a different patient's information written down. When I was in medical school, this was how we kept track of our patients, though it was clear that in residency people used printed-out patient lists. These were the only cards I could picture.

"No, birthday, holiday cards—those types."

Birthday, holiday cards, graduation cards, cards for every occasion she could imagine. Cards for bar and bat mitzvahs. Cards for Halloween. Cards for the next ten years for her son and daughter. Cards so she could be a part of their lives. Cards because she was so proud of them. Cards so she could live those years with them over the course of her last night on earth. Cards so they would never forget her.

I was up for the rest of that night, caring for others and watching her stay up all night, writing, her eyes intent on the cards in front of her, sometimes her husband holding the clipboard, sometimes her friend. As she finished, and as her breathing became more labored, she asked that her morphine dose be increased.

Of course, there were other emergencies. Mr. Wilson's breathing did not get much better even after Dave intubated him, so we had to increase the amount of oxygen and pressure support he received. Mrs. Flannigan passed away at 4 a.m., just after her husband had left her to go home and catch a couple of winks. Throughout my career, I would see the same thing occur, a person dying just a few minutes after his or her spouse had departed, as if giving them one last gift, of sparing them the lasting image of their departure from this earth. Dave walked with me into the room.

"Have you ever pronounced anyone before?" he asked. I admitted that I had not.

"It's easy. Come over here." I walked next to him, by the lifeless body's side. "Lift up her eyelids and shine a light in her eyes, to see if the pupils react." I did what he told me.

It was creepy, touching the dead woman's face. The pupils remained fixed.

"Great. Now check if she's breathing. Put your ear near her mouth and listen, and then listen to her lungs with your stethoscope." Only then did I noticed that the nurse had removed her breathing tube before we came in the room, and had shut off her ventilator. I did what Dave told me to do. Again, nothing. Eerie silence.

"Okay. Now listen with your stethoscope to her heart. You need to listen for one minute without hearing a beat." I watched the second hand on the wall clock make an entire revolution as I listened again with my stethoscope, this time to the heart. A minute is a long time to be crouched over a body that is quickly getting cold to the touch. All for naught. I looked up at Dave and shook my head.

"Great job, champ. You took a life out of this world. Now we just have to work on teaching you to keep them here," he joked. I half smiled, too tired to come up with a snappy response, or to argue. At least I had done one thing right in the past 21 hours.

The sun soon rose over the Charles River. Dave beckoned me to a sink, which had one of those boiling water dispensers you could use to make tea quickly, or even hot cocoa. He turned the handle, and soaked a couple of washcloths under the steaming water. He then wrung them out, handed me one, and placed the other over his face, barbershop style. I did the same. It felt amazing, instantly rejuvenating. We stood with our washcloths by the sink for a minute or two before Janet came up to us.

"Mrs. Abrams just passed. Her husband and friend are in the room."

I looked at Dave hesitantly. I had just learned how to pronounce a person dead, but wasn't sure I could handle this in front of other people. He divined what I was thinking.

"I'll take care of it," he said.

More than two decades have passed, and I still think about Mrs. Abrams and the cards she wrote to her children. The power of her intense fragility—or was it strength? I wonder if I would do the same for my children, now that I have them, or how I would deal with this cache of missives from another world if I were her husband. I also think of her son and daughter—did they look forward to getting these cards every year, or did they dread them? Did they save them? As a parent, I would hope so. But maybe her uncertain handwriting during her final hours reminded her kids of the time when she was sick, so they rejected the cards for earlier, happier memories.

It's rare in life that we can pinpoint one moment that causes a seismic shift in our thinking that leads to our careers veering completely off course from what we imagined. Right then, I decided to become an oncologist. And though I can provide perfectly compelling reasons for my choice—including the fascinating biology of the diagnoses, the opportunities for research, or the prospects for conducting clinical trials of novel drugs—in reality I made the choice so that I could have even a glancing connection to the people who face these terrible cancers with dignity, and in so doing, give value to the lives of everyone around them.

All because of Mrs. Abrams, who wanted to have a say after her death.

The rest of the team straggled in at 7 a.m. My co-interns, especially the guy who was to be on call next, looked horrified at my appearance. He handed me a coffee and a muffin—one of our many traditions—the on-call intern always brought in breakfast for the post-call intern.

"How was it?" he asked, not sure if he wanted to hear the answer. I paused before responding.

"Oh, great!" I said. "Sorry, I'm just a little slow on the uptake right now because of all of the sleep I got."

Dave had been listening in. "That's my boy!" he exclaimed. "Now you're catching on!"

Dave and I checked on our patients and joined the team for rounds with Dr. Thompson, who had so much energy he nearly bounded from one patient to the next. I almost fell asleep, twice, while standing up. We got together for lunch in the conference room and for another teaching session, this time courtesy of the pulmonary/critical care fellow, and then Dave and I were free to go home.

Years later, when I was a hematology/oncology fellow at the Dana-Farber Cancer Institute in Boston, my pager went off, and I saw a number with a Boston area code, but one that was unfamiliar. I called the number, and on the other end of the line I heard Dave's familiar voice. He had become a pulmonary/critical care specialist at another Boston hospital and had just joined their staff. I suspected that Mrs. Abrams and his experience in the intensive care unit had influenced his career choice, too.

"Hey champ! What's cooking?" he asked loudly. There was something forced about the way he said it, though. I asked him how he was doing.

"Not so well, actually. I'm kinda in the hospital, as a patient." He paused, as if he wasn't quite used to saying the next words out loud. "Yeah, I kinda just got diagnosed with lymphoma, and I need to figure out what to do next."

We chatted for a few minutes and I helped arrange for him to see one of the lymphoma specialists where I was training. Things had come full circle, to the point where I was finally able to help Dave. He was treated and cured of his cancer, and even went on to become a nationally prominent medical educator.

I wondered if perhaps that, too, was all part of Mrs. Abrams's plan.

Joan was lying in bed, almost sitting upright, with four or five pillows propping her up. An oxygen mask covered her face. A used breathing tube lay on her bedside table next to some bloodstained gauze. I glanced up at the monitor over her bed, which showed an oxygen saturation of 94 percent. Joan's kids, not as coiffed as in the photo from her room, were there: Her son, a thin guy with closely shaved blond hair, black leather jacket, and a cut-off T-shirt with a marijuana leaf on it, sat in the one chair in the cramped room. Her daughter, who looked to be about 17 and had the same hair color as Joan, stood next to him. She had multiple piercings in each ear and one in her nose. As before, when I saw them in Joan's other hospital room, the worry on their faces belied their hardened appearances.

"How you feeling kiddo?" I asked, loud enough to be heard over the ambient noise. Joan gave me a thumbs-up sign. "I think this is going to be the worst of it," I told her. She locked eyes with me, just as she had prior to being intubated, and nodded, tired. "You made it through. Once the ICU team feels you're stable enough, we'll welcome you back to the leukemia service with open arms," I promised her. The irony, of a leukemia floor being a step in the right direction, escaped neither of us. She mouthed the words "thank you" then closed her eyes and drifted to sleep. I reassured Joan's kids that she was getting better and asked if they had any questions, but they both just shook their heads.

Joan did transfer back to our service later that day. Over the next week and a half, with the help of physical therapy she slowly recovered her strength, and with the help of her healthier bone marrow her blood counts returned to normal. Becky, the resident working with John, discussed her on rounds late one morning.

"I think she's getting better," Becky announced to the team.

"What makes you say that?"

"Well, her white blood cell count is 2,300, which isn't that different from the past few days, but the blasts"—the bad guys—"are gone from her blood stream. And her neutrophils"—the white blood cell subtype that fights bacterial infections—"are over 1,200." Joan had endured the terrible differentiation syndrome brought on by the vitamin A drug, ATRA, but the drug had done its job: the immature blasts had developed into functional neutrophils. With a neutrophil count below 500 or 1,000/μL, Joan was considered "neutropenic" because the quantity of those important neutrophils was considered insufficient to fight life-threatening infections. But with a neutrophil count of 1,200/μL, we considered her immune system competent, and she could potentially go home.

"What about her platelets?" I asked.

"Also normal. She hasn't needed a platelet transfusion in a few days."

"If we discharge her, will her insurance cover the ATRA?" She would need to continue on the drug for another week or two, and intermittently over the next few months. For a vitamin, it was outrageously expensive, at thousands of dollars per month—quite a bit more than the vitamins for sale at our local GNC store—but still a bargain compared to imatinib.

"Yup, her copay isn't bad." Becky reassured me.

"How's she getting around? Is she eating?" I persisted. The basic rules for discharging patients from the hospital include making sure that they can function independently or with minimal assistance at home and sustain themselves nutritionally. Otherwise, we would need to consider a rehabilitation facility.

"She's been walking in the hallway, and she tells me every day that the hospital food is terrible."

"So, you're saying she has insight?" I joked.

The quality (or lack thereof) of hospital food is routinely one of the greatest patient dissatisfiers. Some explanation for this comes from trying to mass-produce meals for 1,400 people at roughly the same time every day—the taste is going to be compromised whether it's at a hospital or a convention. Food also doesn't taste as good because of competing smells, such as those from bleach or other antiseptic interventions required to minimize the spread of germs in the hospital, and from the filtered air on the leukemia floor. Analogously, on an airplane food tastes bland because the dry air at altitude dulls our sense of smell, which compromises our sense of taste.[16] Finally, the drugs we prescribe can change the sense of taste. After receiving chemotherapy, my patients frequently tell me they are more focused on texture than taste, like toddlers. They prefer moist foods, like melons, and can't stand steak or some types of bread. One patient, a former schoolteacher, ate Chinese lo mein for a month because he liked the greasy noodles.

We entered Joan's room. She was sitting at a chair by the window. Her sister Connie, who must have just arrived, was taking off a puffy jacket and slinging it over the back of another chair. Winter was coming, with a dusting of snow forecast for the evening. A bag from Slyman's Deli sat on top of Joan's bedside table, now pulled close to her chair.

"That smells delicious, did you bring enough for all of us?" I asked. Connie smiled.

"I'm going to try the hot pastrami. I usually have the corned beef, but for some reason, it just didn't appeal to me," Joan said.

"I bet that would taste even better in the comfort of your own home."

Joan had been opening the bag from Slyman's and hesitated. "Seriously? I heard rumblings from your posse that I might get out of here. When?" We were a gaggle, but I didn't correct her.

I shrugged my shoulders. "You can finish your sandwich so it doesn't get cold, but any time after that would be fine."

"Is she in a remission?" Connie asked.

"Probably, but we won't know for sure until we perform another bone marrow biopsy, which will happen in a week or so in clinic." Joan had dodged the bullets of infection, bleeding, and differentiation syndrome that kill people with APL during their induction chemotherapy, so she was almost certainly on the good side of the binary outcome, and in a remission.

Joan blinked a couple of times, absorbing the news. Recent events had transpired in a time warp that seemed like a split second and a lifetime all at once: from the moment she sat across the desk from her colleague, the surgeon, who first used the word *leukemia* to describe her condition; to the long drive to Cleveland and her bone marrow biopsy; to watching the red chemotherapy enter her body from the syringe manipulated by Janey's steady hands; to entering the ICU and the horror of the breathing tube (the ICU was a blur, a crazy dream); to the past week of slowly regaining her strength.

Connie started to cry. The enormity of the experience began to hit her too. A golem had attacked her sister—dragging her to that awful ICU for days where she was dehumanized with a breathing tube and multiple intravenous lines, making her use a walker to take just a few steps, and reducing her gustatory range to that of a toddler. But this golem had been defeated, at least temporarily. She rushed over to me and hugged me hard, whispering "thank you" over and over. I hugged her in return, trying to both comfort and reassure. I felt disingenuous at receiving this outpouring of affection.

"All we did was write for chemotherapy and a couple of other drugs. The two of you did all the heavy lifting," I told her and Joan.

"We'll be back to go over your discharge instructions and medications. You'll see us in clinic in a few days," Becky told them, matter-of-factly.

Joan nodded, still stunned, and managed a small smile.

"Home" was all she said.

David Sweeney was the final patient of the day we needed to discuss on rounds. As our gaggle settled back behind our WOWs, Becky updated us on his progress.

"His counts are still in the basement. Whites are 190, hemoglobin 7.8, platelets 7. He's basically requiring either a bag of blood or platelets, or both, every day," she said.

"What day is he?" I asked. We track how long it's been since the first drop of chemotherapy is given (Day 1) to better predict what complications to expect in people with AML, and when their bone marrow will wake up.

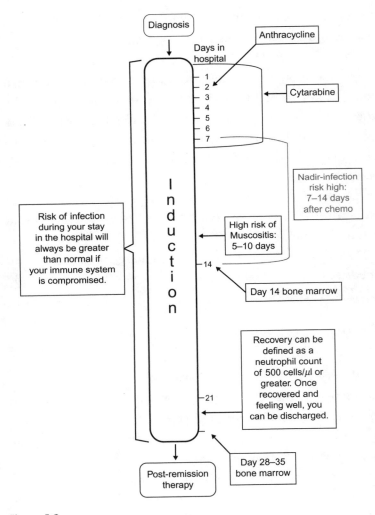

Figure 5.2
The general course of events for a patient with acute myeloid leukemia receiving chemotherapy in the hospital.

The Ara-C finishes infusing on Day 8, the bone marrow biopsy to determine if the leukemia persists occurs on Day 14, and most people recover their blood counts by Day 28, with the first signs of that occurring around Day 21. For those, like David, who need a second course of chemotherapy, it is infused from Days 14 to 19, and blood counts often recover between Days 35 and 42. Bacterial infections can strike at any time, while fungal infections are more likely to hit after Day 10. Breakdown of the tissue linings of the mouth and throat from the chemotherapy (a condition called *mucositis*) occurs in a minority of patients starting around Day 10 or 12, while the same phenomenon can affect the colon around Day 18 (called *neutropenic enterocolitis*). For people with APL receiving ATRA or arsenic, the risk of differentiation syndrome peaks at Days 7 to 10.[17]

"He's Day 27, Day 13 from re-induction chemo," Becky answered.

"Are his fevers gone? How's his diarrhea?" I asked. David, lucky guy that he was, had developed both a fungal infection in his lungs and neutropenic enterocolitis following his terrible bouts of vomiting.

"Tmax 37.8"—his maximum temperature in the past 24 hours, in Celsius, where a temperature of 38, or 100.4 degrees Fahrenheit, is considered febrile—"and he's down to only four or five bowel movements a day. It's better with the immodium." At his worst, he had 10 to 12.

I nodded as I charted all of this in his notes on the computer. Then we went into David's room to see him. He was lying in bed on his side, with the sheets pulled up tight near his head, now bald. The chair by the window was empty. Betty must have gone down to the cafeteria for lunch. He had lost weight, and his cheekbones were more prominent, accentuated by the waxy appearance of his skin. Hard to have much of an appetite on antibiotics and with frequent diarrhea. A bag of packed red blood cells hung on his IV pole, as did IV fluids. I sat down gently at the edge of his bed and lightly placed my hand on his leg.

"David? Hey, sorry to wake you. How are you doing?"

He opened his eyes but wasn't startled. "Groundhog Day," he said softly, alluding to the movie in which Bill Murray plays a weatherman who relives the same day over and over again. One day on the leukemia service can be pretty similar to the next.

"Our goal is to make this as boring a stay as possible for you. Busy night?"

David nodded. "Visited the john a bunch of times. Then the nurse hung the platelets around 6 this morning. She said the counts haven't budged."

"Not yet, but it's still early. I'm hoping to see some signs of life in the next week," I told him.

"God willing," he said. I glanced up to the wall over his bed, where a new plaque hung, decorated with an image of St. Christopher and the words "Protect Us." A couple of angel figurines sat by the window, near the photo of the family tailgating. "He'll get me through this. Through you." David's face was tranquil, without the worry that I had seen a couple of weeks earlier, when I broke the news to him about the persistent leukemia.

Medicine and religion can appear to operate on opposing principles. Whereas most religions are based on faith in an unseen, almighty being, the practice of medicine is empirical. To make a diagnosis, doctors rely on what they observe during an examination (for instance, Joan's petechial rash and persistently bleeding bone marrow biopsy sight indicating low platelets and DIC) and on the supporting laboratory results (a platelet count of 18,000 and abnormal clotting factors).

During my training, my own mentors would go so far as to tell me, "Tumor is a rumor. Tissue is the issue." Even a mass on a CT scan that looks for all the world like cancer isn't called cancer until a piece of it has been removed from the body and examined under a microscope by a pathologist.

There's a joke that emphasizes this principle (and at the same time pokes fun at the priorities of different specialists): Four doctors—an internist, a radiologist, a surgeon, and a pathologist—are out on a boat, duck hunting. They see an object fly across the sky.

Says the internist: "Well, that looks like a duck, but my differential diagnosis for what it could be would include a goose, a hawk, a pterodactyl, and a flying saucer."

The radiologist weighs in: "The image appears to be one of a duck, but I cannot exclude duck-like clouds, scar tissue, or an artifact in how the digital CT scan produces the image."

The surgeon, impatient, grabs a gun, takes aim at the flying object, and shoots it out of the sky. He then scoops it out of the water, hands it to the pathologist, and says, "Tell us what it is."

I struggled for years trying to bring into harmony the factual basis of science and medicine with the faith basis of religion, particularly with what I knew about the bargaining stage of the Kübler-Ross theories, in which an increased focus on religion ("God, if you help me get into remission, I will be a better Christian") might be used as a coping mechanism. I wondered (perhaps unfairly) if that truly represented faith or just desperation, a means to an end.

Then I met a young woman who had endured even more side effects to chemotherapy than David. She retained her generosity of spirit, equanimity, and poise throughout, relying frequently on her faith even when she was at her worst, always pointing out to me that there were others in more need.[18]

Soon after completing her treatment, she and her husband, who were childless, started fostering some at-risk children as a way to give back what she considered the blessing of her good health.

"I've prayed about it," she told me.

When the young woman became pregnant, we celebrated her joy at being able to bring another child, one they had conceived, into their home. But then, during our next appointment, she shared the news she'd learned from her obstetrician just a day earlier: her baby had a rare congenital syndrome that would make it highly unlikely for him to achieve developmental milestones beyond infancy and to live long enough to see his tenth birthday.

I consoled her, as her tears flowed unfettered, and told her what a lucky guy he was to have her as a mother.

She smiled at me, reassuringly. "We'll love him no matter what. It's all part of a greater plan."

Her face became tranquil, just as David's had. With her calm, her strength through such adversity, I finally saw God.

It wasn't until Day 38 that David's neutrophil count—the white blood cells that fight bacterial infections—crested 500, rendering his immune system competent enough to face the outside world. Rachel, Becky, John, and I entered his room to tell him the good news, but Janey must have beaten us there: He was sitting in a chair, dressed, across from Betty, who was also in a chair. The photos, plaque, and figurine were all put away, and his suitcase was packed. Their daughter Susan stood by the window. They were all smiling broadly, though David's expression looked more weathered.

"The team and I took a vote, and we decided you're taking up some bed space that sick people need, so we're politely asking that you leave," I joked.

"We'll take him!" Susan volunteered.

I turned to Betty. "You'll have to clean up all of those beer cans and pizza boxes before David gets home."

"Nah. If I did that, he wouldn't recognize the place," she countered. We all laughed.

"In all seriousness, Janey will go over your medications and follow-up appointments. You have a bunch of them." David could go home because his immune system was recovering, but he still needed blood and platelet transfusions every couple of days. He also needed to continue his antibiotics for the fungal infection. He was far from being out of the woods, and the delay in recovery of his platelet counts nagged at me.

"We'll do whatever it takes to get him outta here," Susan said. "Even if it means an appointment every day, as long as we get him in his own bed every night."

"My own bed." David shook his head, marveling over this most basic of creature comforts denied to him for almost six weeks. Then he looked over to me. "I am grateful, to you and to Him," David said, pointing toward the ceiling.

"Me too," I told him.

6
Things Fall Apart

Turning and turning in the widening gyre
The falcon cannot hear the falconer
   —William Butler Yeats, "The Second Coming," 1920

Joan looked incredible.

A week after leaving the hospital, on a Friday, she was sitting in one of my examination rooms, the same one Sarah, Joe, and Anthony had occupied. Her daughter Courtney sat next to her. They were both laughing as I entered the room, perhaps at a private joke or a funny memory. It was a concrete reminder of how I come into people's lives suddenly, sometimes briefly, sometimes for years, but always for a discrete period, and always as a guest reluctantly invited.

She was wearing a "cranial/hair prosthesis for alopecia." That's the term I have to write on the prescription so the insurance company will cover the cost, I guess because "wig" is too vague. It was the same brown as her hair when I first met her, styled in the same bob. She wore a little foundation and blush, along with eye shadow. But underneath the makeup natural color glowed in her cheeks, that warmth to the skin that we associate with good health. Her recent test results showed that her blood counts had returned to near normal, and her hemoglobin was 12 g/dl, a far cry from the hemoglobin of 7.3 from a month earlier.

Jackie, the outpatient nurse, sat at the desk, so I took a seat on the exam table.

"I didn't notice a wheelchair outside the room. How did you make it here from the car?" I asked.

"Oh, I walked from the front of the building, where Courtney dropped me off."

"She hasn't used a walker in days," Courtney answered, as if this were the most normal thing in the world. The resilience of the human body and spirit, and its ability to recover from the physical and emotional trauma we inflict on it as we try to beat back leukemia, still amazes me. Only 20 days ago, she was in the intensive care unit, on a breathing tube with a guarded diagnosis.

"You've come a long way, Joan," I told her, stating the obvious. She held my gaze and nodded her agreement, co-conspirator that I was in her travails. "And I have some good news about your bone marrow biopsy." She had undergone the procedure a couple of days earlier.

"Jackie already told us! Remission, huh? And who said you can't teach an old surgical nurse new tricks?" Jackie and I laughed. "But the genetic abnormality is still there?"

"Yes, but that's not unusual. Most of the time we still detect the chromosome 15 and 17 translocation after the first course of chemo. It should go away after the arsenic."

Courtney, who had been flipping through screens on her phone, momentarily stopped and looked up. "Arsenic?" she asked. It appeared that we had inadvertently stumbled upon the one word that could penetrate teenage phone screen fixation syndrome, a finding I would be sure to write up for a medical journal for its far-reaching public health implications.

"Yes honey, we talked about this," Joan said to her. "Remember, I told you the biggest side effect to arsenic is its name." Courtney rolled her eyes and went back to her phone.

"Your schedule starts this coming Monday. You'll be here six days a week for the next four weeks. Then we'll take a two-week break and start over," Jackie told her. "Here's your schedule." She handed Joan a calendar marked with the treatment dates and printouts from the electronic medical record with her treatment times.

Joan flipped through the papers. "No rest for the weary."

"No, I'm afraid not. I'm sorry Joan. We'll check an EKG weekly to make sure the arsenic isn't affecting your heart, and of course keep monitoring your blood counts. But you're basically here off and on for the next 10 weeks," I said.

"If that's what we gotta do, let's get started," Joan said, resolved. We said our goodbyes, and Jackie and I went to see our next patient. Courtney followed her mom down the hallway, only occasionally looking up from her phone.

A couple of days later, Rachel was waiting for me in the out-patient clinic hallway by the same exam room door.

"Okay for me to see Mr. Sweeney with you?" she asked.

"Always," I answered. "How do his blood counts look?"

She crinkled her nose. "Not so good. His neutrophil count actually went down, from 500 to 180. And his platelets haven't budged. He needed transfusions every two or three days since being discharged, and he needs them again today."

We knocked on his door and went in. David looked much as he did in the hospital. As opposed to Joan, his skin was still sallow, and what I could see of his arms were covered with bruises and the red spots, called petechiae, that indicate small bleeds under the surface and result from a low platelet count. He was wearing sweatpants and an Ohio State Buckeyes T-shirt, with a blanket draped over his shoulders. Betty was by his side, much as Courtney had been with Joan, but with notebook and pen at the ready. We said our hellos and shook hands all around, as I eased myself onto the exam table once again.

"How have you been, Mr. Sweeney?" Rachel asked.

David shrugged his shoulders. "Okay, I guess. Not much energy."

"How much time are you spending sitting or lying down per day?" Rachel was trying to assess what's called a performance status, a measure of how well a person with cancer functions. There are two major ways to determine it: The Eastern Cooperative Group (ECOG) tool, developed by one of the National Cancer Institute Cooperative groups in 1982 (but based on a previous scale developed in 1960), uses scores on a range from 0 (no impairments) to 5 (death).[1] It always struck me as strange that any performance assessment tool should include death. If a patient is dead, and you need a functional test to assess that, you probably shouldn't be practicing medicine. The Karnofsky scale, named for David Karnofsky, an oncologist at Memorial Sloan Kettering Cancer Center in New York, published in 1949, uses scores on a range from 100 percent (no limitations) to 0 percent (moribund or dead).

Table 6.1
Karnofsky Performance Scale Index (KPS)[2]

Score (category)	Karnofsky
100	Normal; no complaints; no evidence of disease.
90	Able to carry on normal activity; minor signs or symptoms.
80	Normal activity with effort; some signs or symptoms of disease.
70	Care for self but unable to carry on normal activity or do active work.
60	Requires occasional assistance but is able to care for most of his needs.
50	Requires considerable assistance and frequent medical care.
40	Disabled; requires special care and assistance.
30	Severely disabled; hospitalization necessary; active supportive treatment is necessary.
20	Very sick; hospitalization necessary; active supportive treatment is necessary.
10	Moribund; fatal processes progressing rapidly.
0	Dead.

Table 6.2

ECOG Performance Status[3]

ECOG/WHO score system (0–5)	Definition	Karnofsky score
0	Fully active, able to carry on all pre-disease activities without restriction.	90–100
1	Restricted in a physically strenuous activity but ambulatory and able to carry out work of a light or sedentary nature.	70–80
2	Ambulatory and capable of all self-care but unable to carry out any work activities; up and about more than 50% of waking hours.	50–60
3	Capable only of limited self-care, confined to bed or chair 50% or more of waking hours.	30–40
4	Completely disabled; cannot carry on any self-care; totally confined to bed or chair.	10–20
5	Dead.	

ECOG: Eastern Cooperative Oncology Group; WHO: World Health Organization; PS: performance score.

The ways of determining a patient's health are notoriously subjective and can be influenced by a number of factors. A doctor is unlikely to support an aggressive treatment approach, for example, if he or she spies a wheelchair in the hallway outside of an examination room—the assumption being that if a patient needs a wheelchair to get from the car to the clinic, that person may not be able to withstand intensive chemotherapy or invasive surgery.

One colleague of mine demonstrated such biases during a presentation when she showed a slide of an older man in a hospital gown whose wire-rimmed glasses were askew, hair was mussed, and who held a vacant expression. She asked the audience who would treat his leukemia with the same type of 7+3 chemotherapy regimen we gave to David. Nobody raised a hand. She then showed a slide of the same man wearing a natty tie and sports coat with stylish, horn-rimmed glasses at a family gathering. Her family. It was her father-in-law, she admitted. She apologized for lying about his health because he didn't actually have leukemia. Now, how many in the audience would offer him intensive chemo-therapy? People laughed, a bit uncomfortably, at the public revelation of their unconscious biases, and how stereotypes influenced their hypothetical treatment recommendations. The ECOG and Karnofsky systems are an attempt to stan-dardize such assessments using objective criteria.

David shrugged his shoulders again as Betty answered for him. "He goes to bed around 8 at night and sleeps for about 10 to 12 hours. During the day, he spends most of his time on the couch, and he naps a bit during the afternoon." That would translate to an ECOG performance status score of 3. He wasn't doing too well.

"That's not true Bet. I get up and do things," David snapped at her, annoyed. It was the first time I had seen any tension between them. How frustrating it must have been for him, someone who held a factory job, provided for his family, and raised two kids, to have spent so much time in the hospital and actually feel worse than when he started. Betty pursed her lips, but didn't respond.

"Any fevers?" Rachel continued. David shook his head. "Bleeding?"

David pulled up his sleeves to show us the ecchymotic, bruised and darkened terrain of his forearms. "I can't really brush my teeth, either. My gums are a mess, they bleed every time."

"Are you eating and drinking?"

David shrugged his shoulders a third time. "Food's better than in the hospital, but I just don't have an appetite." Probably a combination of the anemia and the multiple pills (including antibiotics) he still had to take as we awaited the full recovery of his immune system—as well as what might be a low-grade depression. "But I am drinking a couple of those hospital cups full of water a day." The cups are a parting gift when people are discharged—each holds 32 ounces of fluid—so he was doing well with hydration.

"You do need a blood transfusion today. And platelets," Rachel told him. "Those will take you through the weekend."

Betty nodded. "We figured as much." She wrote this information down in "The Book of David."

"I wonder if we should think about another bone marrow biopsy, too," I added. Betty glanced up toward me, and then wrote "bone marrow biopsy" in the notebook. The day's date was at the top of the page.

"Okay," she said slowly. "Why's that?"

"I was hoping to see the blood counts improve a bit more since you've been home. But you're still requiring a lot of transfusions, and the neutrophils have slipped. It's possible the bone marrow is still just wiped out from all the chemo we gave you, and is taking its own, sweet time to recover. Or . . ."

"Or the leukemia never went away." David finished my thought. The golem in the room. That damn golem, always lurking in one of my examination rooms.

I nodded. "I just can't tell based on your blood counts, and I've seen both scenarios play out: people whose bone marrows take a while to recover and are alive years later; and people with blood counts like yours because they still have leukemia. Let's figure out what's going on and we'll have a plan either way."

Betty underlined "bone marrow biopsy" in the notebook but didn't say anything else. David adjusted the blanket covering his shoulders, wrapping it tighter.

The following Monday, Day 15 of her treatment cycle, Joan was getting her arsenic. The colorless, odorless, and thus ideal poison hung innocently in a clear plastic bag from an IV pole by her infusion chair but, vigilant nurse to the core, only after she had asked to verify the label for its contents—arsenic trioxide injection 10 mg/10 ml.[4] She shook her head, thinking of the paths that led to this moment in her life, staring out the tinted windows to the grassy plaza below. Her hopes were now tied to the drug more notoriously associated with people who want to kill their enemies. Or, as in

Arsenic and Old Lace, Joseph Kesselring's satirical play from the 1940s, with the crazy Brewster sisters, the spinsters who find it their duty to kill "lonely old men" and "help them find peace."[5] Well then, Joan would let arsenic help *her* find peace by similarly dealing with the leukemia.

At the same time, David lay prone on the unyielding bone marrow biopsy table, his pants pulled down to plumber's crack level and his shirt hiked up to the bottom of his ribs. He had already received a transfusion of the straw-colored platelets, to minimize bleeding from the procedure. He had also taken the Percocet and lorazepam—a benzodiazepine also used to help prevent withdrawal in alcoholics—that would both numb the pain and make him care less about any pain he did feel. Next came the deep shot of lidocaine to numb the bone. "Like a bee sting," the physician's assistant told him. Like a lot of bee stings, David thought. Then he heard the motor of the drill turn on, the physician assistant's gloved hand on the small of his back, and the pressure on his pelvis, pushing down . . .

Pushing down . . .

Pushing . . .

"Mr. Sweeney?" He heard his name being called, from far away.

"Mr. Sweeney?" Then closer, and someone shook his shoulder. "We're all done. You fell asleep. Mr. Sweeney?" He pushed himself up and shifted, to lie on his side. Then he sat up. Dizzy.

"Careful buddy!" The physician's assistant held both of his shoulders. "I'll walk you to a chair, and you can pull your pants up all the way. He stood, slowly, and hobbled over to the tan chair near the desk as he yanked his jeans over his newly bandaged posterior. When had this old man taken over his body, his ability to think clearly, his motivation? He sat, arms lax by his side, hands gripping his knees, for Betty to come get him, the old man waiting at the bus stop. *The Old Man and the Sea.* He had read that in school. The old man.

"Hello, it's Karl." I knew it was Karl. He had paged me to his number with his name following the digits, so I had called him. And he never paged to let me know that a bone marrow biopsy was perfectly normal.

"I hesitated to return your page, Karl," I told him. Silence. He knew. He knew how much I liked him, respected him, and admired his skill and dedication. And he knew that he was often the purveyor of bad news—to me—so that I then became the emissary of bad news to another. That person, in turn, would become the carrier of bad news to his or her family. And so the ripples of heartache would continue.

"Mr. Sweeney had a bone marrow biopsy yesterday?" Karl asked. Preparing me for bad news, just as I would prepare the Sweeneys.

"Yup."

Silence, and then, "I count 58 percent blasts. I'm sorry." I knew he was sorry; he didn't have to say it. He hated this part of his job, just as I did. The leukemia had never gone away.

"Thanks for letting me know so quickly," I told Karl. "It means a lot." I didn't have to say that last bit. He knew that too.

The next afternoon, David was in the room. So was Betty. So were Susan and Eric. Rachel had come with me, as had Jackie. More people than chairs. They suspected. In truth, it's rare that I surprise my patients with the news that leukemia persists, or that it has returned. Either they recognize the symptoms that started them on the path to that first diagnosis (the fatigue, the shortness of breath, the bleeding), or they realize that to go so long without achieving a modicum of normalcy, of feeling like they did a year ago, before *leukemia* was part of the daily lexicon, cannot be a good thing.

David and Betty sat in the thin armchairs, Susan on the exam table, and Eric stood by the wall, arms by his side. I sat on the open stool, and rolled it closer to David. Although I have seen some colleagues engage in small talk with patients before conveying bad news, I always felt that was a bit forced, even cruel.[6] We all knew why we were here, and what information David was waiting for.

"David, we sent you for a bone marrow biopsy on Monday because we were worried about your low blood counts, that they hadn't yet recovered, and were even a bit worse than when we discharged you from the hospital. We talked about two reasons why your blood counts could be low: either as a continued side effect of the chemotherapy we gave you, or because the leukemia remained in your bone marrow."

Preparing him. "I got a call from one of our pathologists yesterday afternoon. I'm sorry, but the leukemia is still in your bone marrow. The chemotherapy didn't get rid of it. We weren't able to get rid of it."

David held my gaze for a couple of seconds, and then lowered his eyes to his hands clasped in his lap. Betty gripped her notebook and pen with one hand, and reached over and held David's hands with the other. Susan took a deep breath and sighed.

"We guessed that's what was going on," Betty said quietly.

"How much?" David asked. He wanted a number to compare.

"58 percent blasts," I said simply.

Betty wrote the number in "The Book of David" after jotting the date at the top of the page. On the opposite page, two days earlier, she had written and underlined the words "bone marrow biopsy." One page fear, the other finality. "On Monday you said there would be a plan of what to do either way. What is the plan now that we know the leukemia is still there?"

"Yeah, what treatment can Dad get next?" Eric asked from across the room.

"You have a couple of options," I said to David. "The first would involve your heading back into the hospital to receive chemotherapy. Similar to the 7+3 in intensity, but different chemotherapy and more of it."

"There's no way I'm going back in that place," David said, his jaw set and eyes resolute. "No way. No."

"Dad, why don't you just listen to what the doctor has to say before you make up your mind?" Eric said. "Maybe it won't be as bad."

Rachel looked intently at David, then at Eric, and back to David. He hadn't wanted to receive the intensive, inpatient chemotherapy to start with, but had capitulated to both the spoken and intimated wishes of his family. She hesitated, struggling with whether to intervene more forcefully this time, or continue to let the family figure it out. Sometimes the most powerful tool in communication is to not say anything at all, to give people the space to make their own decisions.

"But he didn't want the aggressive chemotherapy to start with," Rachel said, frustrated. Or, she could take that approach.

Eric glared at her, and Susan squirmed in her place on the exam table.

"The chance that the intensive chemotherapy we would give you in the hospital would work is, at best, half of what I quoted you when we started treating your leukemia," I explained to them. "So, no higher than a 25 percent chance of going into remission, probably less than 20 percent, since we've had such a hard time getting rid of it to start with."

Betty wrote down the number.

I continued. "Unfortunately, the chance that more of the intensive chemotherapy could harm you, or even cause you to die, doesn't decrease, and may be even higher, because of what you've already been through, say 15 to 20 percent."

Betty wrote down that number too, then did a bit of a double take, noticing it was the same percentage as the chance for remission. "And how long would he be in?"

"About the same amount of time as before, a month or more," I answered.

David shook his head. "So it's the same number, alive or dead, and I spend the rest of my time in a hospital bed? What's option B?"

"Dad, that isn't what the doctor said," Susan piped up. "It's an 80 percent chance you'll be alive, but only 20 percent chance you'll get a remission, or 20 percent chance you . . ." She trailed off. But "20 percent chance you don't make it" hung in the air without her having to say it.

"Option B involves some of the genetic tests we sent on your bone marrow sample, when we looked to see if we could find an abnormality that caused your leukemia to occur. Remember, these are not genetic abnormalities that are passed down to Eric or Susan, these arose just in you to cause your bone marrow cells to become cancerous."

David and Betty nodded their understanding and glanced at Rachel, recalling a conversation she had with them weeks ago, similar to the one I had with Joan and her friend Patty.

"Well, your cells had a mutation in what's called *IDH2*— isocitrate dehydrogenase 2. It's involved in some of the cell's metabolic processes that affect its ability to mature. The FDA approved a drug—a pill—that inhibits the mutation, allowing the cell to grow and mature normally again. Only about 10 to 15 percent of people with AML have the mutation.

Which translates to about one out of a million people in the United States."

"Do I have to be treated in the hospital?" David asked.

"That's the good news. It's all outpatient, but we'd have to see you a couple times a week to watch for side effects."

"Such as?" Betty asked, pen poised over the notebook.

Aside from the typical side effects that occur with any drug I use to treat leukemia, which involve worsening the blood counts before potentially improving them, the *IDH2* inhibitor could also cause the differentiation syndrome, similar to the ATRA we used to treat Joan. One FDA report even put the rate of that occurring at almost 20 percent. I explained this to David and his family.[7]

"What's the chance it'll work?" Eric asked.

"In the study that got it approved, about 175 people with leukemia who never entered a remission or relapsed after being in a remission were treated with the drug. Among them, approximately 25 percent went into a remission, and that remission lasted about eight months, on average. Some more, and some less."[8]

"Eight months is good Daddy," Susan said.

Betty wrote, and Rachel nodded to herself as she recalled discussing the study at a recent journal club, one of many regular meetings she and the other hematology-oncology fellows attended as part of their developing skills for research and how to read the medical literature critically.

"Could he get a bone marrow transplant if he goes into a remission?" Eric asked. This time, Rachel rolled her eyes at him.

"From that study, 10 percent of patients—and most of those patients did go into a remission—went on to get a bone marrow transplant. The inhibitor isn't curative, but a bone marrow transplant, where you get a bone marrow from a healthy donor without leukemia, has that potential," I answered.

"Have YOU seen it work?" David asked me, pointedly. He wasn't one for abstract trial results.

"I have. We enrolled 15 patients onto that study, and it worked in a few. One for more than a year and counting," I told him. "But it also didn't work in a few."

David was a straight shooter, and I added this last part not to be harsh, but to let him know I wasn't trying to sell him on a therapy. He wanted the good, the bad, and the ugly.

"What's option C?" he asked.

I exhaled before answering. "David, none of us has gone through what you just endured. And I know you debated at first whether you wanted to get treated at all."

Eric crossed his arms in front of his chest and looked down at the floor, anticipating where I was heading.

"So the option of not treating the leukemia with more chemotherapy, and just taking transfusions when you need them, or not even that, is still on the table. I think it's as valid a choice as the other two." David stared at me, unblinking. "And I will continue to be 100 percent supportive of any choice you make," I added.

"When do I need to decide?"

"There's no rush, but I also don't want you to drive yourself crazy debating this. Why don't you give yourself until the end of the weekend," I offered.

"That's reasonable," he said, even smiling a bit at the irony of the statement. It was neither reasonable that he had leukemia nor that it had proved so particularly recalcitrant to therapy. And now he had to make a decision given the terrible odds with each scenario? There was nothing reasonable about any of this, as both he and I and everyone in the room knew. Reasonable left town about eight weeks ago.

I exited the room with Rachel and we walked back through the heavy glass doors leading to our workroom. It was normally busy, and loud. Nurses, pharmacists, social workers, and doctors sat at the 16 computers lining the outside walls, and along a dividing wall down the middle. Some were reviewing labs, writing orders, or typing patient notes. Others were on the phones with the scheduling personnel trying to squeeze in patients for transfusions or treatments, or with consultants trying to arrange appointments or to get help in treating an infection or managing a patient's cardiac problems. Some spoke with each other, sometimes heatedly, about a patient they were scheduled to see or had just seen, concerning the best course of action to treat that person's cancer. Or more commonly, they discussed the best course given what the patient's insurance would pay for, or what the patient could afford out of pocket.

Similar to the inpatient hospital rooms, these walls were also adorned with mementos from patients past and present:

photos, usually of a patient flanked by his or her doctor and nurse, or of babies born after the chemo was all done; artwork by patients, or their children or grandchildren. On one wall hung a vestigial light box to display hard copies of X-rays, just like it's done in movies or TV shows set in hospitals—only now the X-ray viewing is done on the computer. These mementos reminded us about the people behind the notes and computer data: those we had saved, and others we had lost. Gone but not forgotten.

That afternoon the room was empty, and Rachel and I sat down by the computer I usually used, which was surrounded by plastic toys. A few years earlier, the child of one of our patients had left a toy dragon in an examination room. For reasons that still escape me, one of our rooming nurses assumed it was mine, and placed it in the workroom by my computer. From that point on, in a plotline that could have come straight from the classic sitcoms *The Office* and *Seinfeld*, abandoned superhero or animal figurines found a new home by my computer. Occasionally I'd find the remnants of a pitched battle that one of my coworker's had staged between the plastic warriors, presumably with one side representing the evil leukemia and the other upholding the forces of good chemotherapy. Chemo was always victorious in these fantasy wars. New characters for these vicarious reenactments arrive far less frequently now, as kids more commonly accompany their parents or grandparents to appointments wielding a Nintendo Switch or an iPhone rather than dinosaurs and dolls.

"Can we talk about Mr. Sweeney's son?" I asked.

Rachel took a deep breath. "He drives me crazy. He keeps pushing Mr. Sweeney to get more chemotherapy, to keep treating his leukemia. He just spent six weeks in the hospital, when he didn't even want to be there in the first place. And it was a waste of time—the chemo didn't work. Why can't he see how beat up his father is?"

"Well . . . because it's his father," I said softly. A decade earlier, I would have reacted the same way as Rachel. Part and parcel with the doctor-patient relationship, we're trained (somewhat paternalistically or maternalistically) to be protective of our patients. Naturally, we want to safeguard their physical health, but also their emotional well-being, and we try to face down threats to either. Rachel saw Eric as a threat.

But then my own father died, suddenly. In what my mother described as every wife's worst nightmare, she came home from work one evening in late January to find him collapsed on the kitchen floor, by the chair he always occupied to read the newspaper. He had probably suffered a cardiac arrest. Being a notorious spendthrift who kept the house's temperature in the low 60s in the dead of the Rhode Island winter, he had turned on an electric space heater nearby as he perused the local news, and luckily the heater had not overturned when he fell.

"His face was still warm," my mother said, over and over again. The heater had cycled on and off by his body throughout that day. Therefore, he couldn't be dead, right?

I had a hard time believing it myself. Regardless of our relationship with them, our parents represent an element of our core truth. When one parent dies, a part of that truth dies too. Confronting our own mortality is hard; facing a parent's is no easier. A child's—I couldn't imagine. Eric's truth was being threatened, so he was doing what he could to protect it, even at the expense of what may have been his father's needs.

I elaborated on this with Rachel. "You're right, that our primary responsibility is always to our patient. Part of that obligation is also to tend to the needs of the people who are important to our patient."

"And if those needs are in conflict?" she asked.

"We try to reach consensus within the room. If that can't happen, it's okay to identify the differing opinions, and to say out loud that you're having trouble rectifying what you're hearing are the desires of your patient, with those of a family member. It's also okay to be transparent with the family about where your responsibility lies. In almost every situation, even with difficult decisions like the one Mr. Sweeney is facing, families will respect a patient's choice. Give them time." Rachel nodded. "And try not to antagonize anyone. Or roll your eyes." I added, smiling at her. "Look at it from Eric's perspective. He doesn't want his dad to die."

"I know," she said, thinking about the interaction. "I just don't like him."

My own idealism about liking (or even feeling comfortable around) every one of my patients was shattered during my residency. A man was admitted to our hospital service from jail, with a new diagnosis of lung cancer. I entered his room to take his history and perform a physical exam and found him sleeping, still wearing his orange jumpsuit, with one leg cuffed to the bed's footboard. Two prison guards stood nearby. I went over to the bed and touched the man's shoulder gently, and he startled awake. Never will I forget how those clear blue eyes stared right through me, with hate. Every fiber in my body stood at alert, as danger—real and in the flesh—faced me down. When I was through, which didn't take long, given his monosyllabic answers and my mounting fear, I left the room. One of the guards followed me out.

"Hey doc," he said. "Not for nothin' . . . but don't ever wake one of these guys by shaking his shoulder. They're used to being attacked in jail, and you're lucky he didn't clobber you. You gotta get a stick"—with that he removed a billy club from his belt—"and whack him in the feet." He hit the hospital wall with the club.

I thanked him for the advice, uncertain whether he was having fun by intimidating me, or if he was just plain putting me on—but wondering nevertheless if he were serious. Would a reflex hammer, or even a gentle shaking of the foot, also do the trick?

"Can I ask what was he in for?" I did, in fact, ask. You can usually pick out the healthcare worker in the room by observing who asks permission to ask a question.

The guard leaned toward me and spoke in a lower voice. "He murdered his wife. With a hammer."

I shivered in the hospital hallway. I did not like this man. In fact, he frightened me. But I cared for him as I would anyone else, albeit without the hug at the end of his hospital stay.

"You're not going to like every patient, or every family member. Me neither, and it's okay to admit that. But we both have to care for them, without prejudice, nonetheless," I said to Rachel. We then talked about the impact this can have on healthcare providers. Few other professions come with the expectation that you will willingly place yourself in a situation where you can be vulnerable to either physical or psychological harm, every day. Some have even linked this expectation to the higher rates of burnout among doctors and nurses.[9]

"How's Joan Walker doing?" I asked as I turned to the computer to pull up her labs.

"Fine, I think. She may be differentiating again," Rachel said.

"What do you mean? She's already differentiated. That's what landed her in the ICU after we started her on induction chemotherapy in the hospital." Joan's white blood cells had already matured and become normal after she received the ATRA along with the chemo. It would be pretty unusual for it to happen while receiving arsenic for two weeks.

"Well, she has a lot of white cells at various stages of maturation in her blood, and also blasts again," Rachel said, less sure this time.

The numbers I saw on the computer confused me. Joan's blood counts would be expected to be a bit abnormal from the arsenic, but not to the levels that were being flagged in her chart: hemoglobin of 7.2, platelet count of 68,000, and white blood cell count that had ballooned to 45,000—closer to when she was diagnosed than to when she was discharged from the hospital. The subtypes of white blood cells were listed, and there, at the bottom of the screen, was the most worrisome lab value of all: blasts at 25 percent.

"Oh no" was all I could say. I stared at the screen, trying to will the numbers to normalize. Rachel looked at me, then at the computer, then back to me. Rare for the leukemia to differentiate at this point due to the arsenic, just as rare for it to relapse despite the arsenic. Blasts . . . 25 percent. High white blood cell count. Low platelets and hemoglobin. The indifferent computer screen wasn't lying. Her leukemia had come raging back.

"What do we do?" Rachel asked.

I pulled my eyes away from the golem's bloody evidence. "We tell Joan."

We left the workroom and hoofed it over to the infusion area. Jackie met us halfway there.

"You saw her labs?" Jackie asked, staring at the worry on my face. I frowned and nodded. "I'll schedule the hospital admission after you tell her," she said. "She doesn't feel well."

I carried the news of a patient's relapsed leukemia like a millstone around my neck, my body aching with the burden of privileged, awful information not yet imparted. Rachel, Jackie, and I paused outside her room, gathering strength for what was about to happen, for the seismic shift that would occur as she moved from the path to recovery (and a possible cure) to an uncertain future. I knocked at her door and we all entered.

Joan was in the blue infusion chair, reclined at a La-Z-Boy angle. Her sister Connie sat in the single, thin-armed chair by the window. It looked like the clear arsenic had just dripped in for the day. I greeted both of them.

"You're here with reinforcements, I don't feel well, and I don't like the look on your face," Joan said. "I also haven't seen the printout of my labs yet. The past two weeks, I've seen them by the time the arsenic is done." She was so damn observant.

Jackie handed her the printout as I started to speak. "Joan, your labs are pretty abnormal. After you were discharged from the hospital, your blood counts seemed to be recovering, and your bone marrow results looked fine."

"But the genetic abnormality was still there," she said, almost to herself. "So the leukemia probably hadn't gone away." She was right. I had told her it was "not unusual" to retain the chromosome 15 and 17 translocation after the intensive chemotherapy course. I had even used the double negative to explain it to her, another favorite among health-care providers when the answer is not absolute. The vast majority of the time those abnormalities would disappear after more therapy with the arsenic. But infrequently, persistence of the genetic translocation could also be abnormal, a sign that the golem was plotting his return.

She continued to look over the lab printout. "And now I have 25 percent blasts. It's back. The leukemia's back. No wonder I feel like crap."

"Is that true? Has Joan's leukemia returned?" Connie asked, looking first at Joan, and then at me and Jackie.

I nodded. "I'm sorry. It has. We'll run tests on the blasts in Joan's blood to confirm, but in the meantime we'll arrange for another stay in the hospital and more chemotherapy. We have a really good chance of getting this back into remission." I held Joan's gaze and nodded my head a couple of times. *Trust me. You can do this again. This isn't all for naught. We haven't given up on you, so don't give up on yourself.* "And then we would plan for a bone marrow transplant to make sure we get rid of the leukemia for good."

"What does that involve?" Connie wondered.

The science behind bone marrow transplantation, and the series of events that led to its routine use in disorders like leukemia, is remarkable.

The basic concept seems straightforward: We are limited in the amount of chemotherapy we can use to treat cancers because of the side effects of the chemotherapy. If we could only give more chemo, we could cure a person of leukemia. If we did that, though, we would be facing what I have heard colleagues derisively refer to as a "Harvard death": the leukemia would be gone (thus, the treatment was technically successful), but the patient would be dead.

The major dose-limiting side effect of chemotherapy used to treat leukemia is bone marrow suppression. During the weeks David and Joan spent in the hospital when their blood counts were low, they were highly susceptible to life-threatening infections, and they needed blood and platelet transfusions regularly. If we were to give patients like them even more chemotherapy, the bone marrow would never regenerate, and the immune system, red blood cells, and

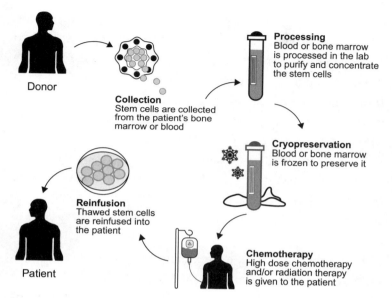

Figure 6.1
The general process of bone marrow transplantation.

platelets would never recover; they would die from an infection or would bleed to death.

But what if we could rescue the bone marrow that was obliterated by chemotherapy by replacing it with healthy bone marrow?

There are two ways this can be accomplished. The first is called an *autologous* bone marrow transplant.[10] It involves harvesting the bone marrow from a person with cancer, which in itself can be done in several ways—either by performing multiple bone marrow biopsies, or by giving the person drugs that cause the bone marrow to "mobilize" its cells into the blood stream, then collecting those bone marrow cells from a large IV in a vein, through a process called *apheresis*, and storing it. Next, that person is given whopping doses of chemotherapy to annihilate the cancer, and then that same person's stored bone marrow is reinfused after the chemotherapy has wiped out the bone marrow (and hopefully any remaining cancer in that person's body).

The second is called an *allogeneic* bone marrow transplant. It requires harvesting bone marrow from a person who doesn't have the cancer, and infusing that bone marrow into the cancer patient who has received the whopping dose of chemotherapy.

Both have been used to treat leukemia. The problem with an autologous transplant in someone with leukemia is that it's almost impossible to ensure that the re-transplanted bone marrow—even after it has gone through a "cleaning" process to remove cancerous cells—doesn't stubbornly retain the original leukemia. Studies that compare performing autologous transplants on leukemia patients to just giving them more standard chemotherapy treatments have found that patients live just as long with either approach.

Autologous bone marrows also lack one of the most important factors in curing leukemia: the transplantation of another person's immune system to attack and destroy any remaining leukemia cells in the recipient's body.

The first successful bone marrow transplant from one human to another human with leukemia took place in 1959 in Cooperstown, New York. The donor and recipient were identical twins. Dr. E. Donnall Thomas, who performed the procedure, went on to win the Nobel Prize in physiology or medicine in 1990 along with Dr. Joseph E. Murray, who pioneered kidney transplantation. Dr. Thomas had been drawn to the identical twins because they shared the same genetics: the chance that one twin would react to or reject the other's bone marrow was low.

Prior to the twin transplant, as shown by studies published in 1950 and conducted in the classified laboratories of the Atomic Energy Commission in Rochester, New York, dogs had been given high doses of radiation to destroy their marrows, and then had been infused with marrows from other dogs. But those transplants failed; the dogs had died. Subsequent studies in mice, however, found that if a mouse "accepted" a transplanted bone marrow from another mouse, it would also accept a skin graft from that same mouse—indicating that donor bone marrow cells could successfully be transferred.

Thomas carried out similar experiments in dogs—beagles, to be specific—and was able to demonstrate in successful autologous transplants that bone marrow cells could be obtained from the blood stream, and that the cells could be stored for periods of time before being reinfused.[11] He had pledged to himself that if the transplants were successful, he would care for the transplanted dogs for the rest of their lives. Eventually, with dozens of dogs living in his backyard, he suddenly realized he was on to something big—and that he would have to start sending some of the dogs to be fostered by other families!

As a next step, he infused donor marrow into patients and demonstrated that it was possible for another's marrow to take up residence in a recipient's bone, and that this could be done with an intravenous infusion. This is an aspect of transplantation that still amazes me: bone marrow, infused just as we would a bag of blood, can flow through the veins and arteries and somehow retain the ability not only to find the bone marrow space, but also set up shop there.

This first transplant performed by Thomas, between genetically identical people, is referred to as a *syngeneic* transplant. Although it's probably more effective than an autologous transplant in a person with leukemia because it avoids the problem of a marrow still contaminated with cancer, we now recognize that it isn't ideal, as identical twins also share identical immune systems.

The bone marrow transplant in Thomas's twins was successful in two ways: (1) it was not rejected; and (2) the twin with leukemia recovered his blood counts afterward. But his leukemia came raging back within a few months, as might have been predicted with a syngeneic transplant: the transplanted immune system, being genetically identical to his own, would not recognize the remaining leukemia cells as "foreign" and thus would not trigger the immune system to attack and destroy those cells. In addition, his own leukemia probably hadn't been sufficiently eliminated at the start (before the transplant) by radiation, the method used for decades as a "preparative regimen" to kill the leukemia-containing bone marrow.

Transplants from one of Thomas's beagles to another mostly failed, either because the transferred marrow didn't stick, or when it did, the new immune system attacked the recipient's body. But an occasional dog, with a littermate bone marrow donor, went through the procedure well, and went on to have a normal lifespan.

The littermate bone marrow donor—that was the key.

Scientists began to recognize that non-twins could be a "match" for each other if they shared some of the same proteins on the surface of cells that were responsible for regulation of the immune system. These proteins are encoded by genes known as the human leukocyte antigen (HLA) complex, located on chromosome 6. Once techniques were developed to assess HLA genes, it became straightforward, Mendelian-type genetics: siblings who share the same parents (inheriting half their genetic material from each parent) have a 25 percent chance of being HLA identical, and thus capable of being bone marrow donors for each other.

These were the compatible beagle littermates.

The first non-twin transplant took place in Minnesota in 1968, performed by Dr. Robert Good, and involved a sibling who donated bone marrow to an infant with a congenital immunodeficiency disorder. The first bone marrow transplant between unrelated people occurred in 1973, in New York, when a boy who was born with an immunodeficiency disease received multiple transplants from a donor in Denmark.[12]

But how to get around the issue of an immune system intolerant of a non-genetically identical transplanted bone marrow, or the opposite—the transplanted bone marrow, and thus transplanted immune system—that won't tolerate the body into which it is transplanted?

The success of non-twin transplants could not have occurred without the development and use of immuno-suppressive drugs, such as methotrexate, cyclosporine, and immuran. These drugs prevented the recipient (or *host*) from rejecting the new bone marrow (the *graft*), but also pre-vented the transplanted immune system produced by the new bone marrow from attacking the host's vital organs.[13]

That's the trick, actually: to allow the transplanted immune system to be active enough to attack and eliminate any residual leukemia, but not so active that it attacks and eliminates, say, the liver or the intestines, a phenomenon known as *graft versus host disease* (GVHD). In patients who had undergone bone marrow transplants for leukemia in the 1970s, in fact, those who had some GVHD were less likely to have leukemia that returned compared to those who had no GVHD. It was recognized that the transplanted immune system probably played a greater role in eliminating leftover leukemia than the high doses of radiation or chemotherapy given to patients prior to the transplant.

A series of elegant dog experiments by Dr. Ranier Storb and his colleagues at the Fred Hutchinson Cancer Research Center in Seattle, Washington, then showed that the amount of chemotherapy or radiation given as a preparative regimen prior to the bone marrow transplant could be reduced if the amount of immunosuppressive drug dose were raised.[14] This allowed for transplants to be given without completely wiping out the recipient's bone marrow—paving the way for *reduced intensity* transplants in older adults who couldn't tolerate the previous toxic preparative regimens.

The latest advances in bone marrow transplantation have included the use of umbilical cord blood from newborns, which is rich in the stem cells normally found in the bone marrow, and the use of what are called haploidentical transplants, in which the bone marrow donor is only half a genetic match to the person with leukemia—as would occur with a child donating marrow to a parent.[15]

Umbilical cord blood transplantation started in 1988, with cord blood from a sibling that was processed in Indiana and hand delivered in a cooler to an infant in France who had an inherited anemia. That infant was still alive decades later. Since then, tens of thousands of cord transplants have been performed.

Haploidentical bone marrow transplants were first attempted in the 1980s, but without much success, due to high rates of severe GVHD. With the donor immune system being so different from the recipient, it was inevitable that it would attack the recipient's vital organs. But with advances in GVHD prevention, both by manipulating the transplanted bone marrow and through immunosuppressive therapy, these types of transplants have become much more common, with more than a 1,000 "mismatched" transplants performed each year.[16]

Though the following claim is an exaggeration, I have overheard some transplant specialists say that there's almost no such thing as someone who *can't* find a bone marrow match anymore.

I explained the concept underlying bone marrow transplants to Connie and Joan.

"Our first step will be to see if Connie is a genetic match for you, which we would do through a simple blood sample. As I mentioned, there's only a 25 percent chance that she will be, so if not, we would then go through the Be The Match program, where a transplant team can go to search (on behalf of a patient needing a transplant) for a genetically similar stranger who is registered in its database as a willing donor—a relationship I have heard referred to as a "brother from another mother" or a "sister from another mister." Joan was white, so the chance she would find an unrelated bone marrow donor through Be The Match was greater than 75 percent. If she were African American or black, the chance would shrink to less than 25 percent—the lowest likelihood among the ethnic groups the program provides comparative data for on its website—because of genetic complexity in people of certain races, and fewer available donors.[17]

Connie looked away while we were having this conversation. I imagine it must have been tough for her, knowing that the odds she could save her sister's life by giving Joan her bone marrow were less than those for the flip of a coin. The cruelty of genetic randomness.

Joan asked us if she could have the weekend to collect her thoughts and get her head wrapped around the latest in a series of her new realities. We scheduled her readmission to the hospital for Monday.

Jackie, Rachel, and I slouched toward the workroom, feeling like the second comings of cancer's return. Leaving chaos in our wake, deflated, ineffectual, and sad. True, we hadn't given David and Joan their cancers. But we hadn't gotten rid of them particularly well, either.

Monday again.

Joan returned to the hospital and stood by Angela's desk at the entrance to the leukemia floor, with Connie by her side. Same black bag, same red yarn identifying it as hers. Same wristband, same leukemia.

Janey spotted her and, without words, walked up and gave Joan a lingering hug.

"Let's get you settled honey," Janey said to Joan. "And let's get you better."

Different room this time, facing east toward the Cleveland Museum of Art, Severance Hall (home of the Cleveland Orchestra), Cleveland Heights, and Shaker Heights, where I lived. Connie helped unpack her bag and put the few clothes she brought into the narrow closet and drawers.

Different residents and interns, too. Becky and John had moved on to other rotations after their four-week stint on the leukemia floor, neither destined for a career in hematology/oncology. An intern in a freshly dry-cleaned shirt was asking Joan a number of questions about her leukemia and how it was being treated; he was typing the information into the computer on his WOW when Jackie and I entered the room, having walked over from clinic. Routine now for Joan, anything but routine to this new guy. I apologized for interrupting.

"Glad you made it in okay, Joan. How was your weekend?"

"Great," Joan answered, smiling. "Saw some friends on Saturday, went out to breakfast with the kids Sunday. It was all so . . . normal," she said, thinking through the events of the past couple of days, and sounding almost surprised that normal had triumphed over abnormal. "I'm ready to get started again."

We chatted for a couple of minutes about what the next few days held in store. We had started to say our goodbyes when Connie stopped us.

"Any chance I could talk to you for a moment in private?" she asked.

Jackie and I left the hospital room with her and walked down the hallway to an empty conference room. We sat down at the table, Connie at the head, Jackie and I at either side.

"About the bone marrow transplant. You need to get a blood sample from me to see if I'm a match for her, right?" Connie asked.

"Right. Like we said, as Joan's sister there's a 25 percent chance your DNA—your genes—are similar enough to hers that you could donate your bone marrow to her, so we check your blood before we go to strangers through the Be The Match program."

Connie shook her head and closed her eyes. "I don't want you to check my blood."

I was surprised. "Oh. Okay. Can I ask why? (Another question requesting permission to ask a question.) Do you not like needles? Or is it because you don't think Joan should undergo a bone marrow transplant?"

"It's because I'm not her sister," she said.

I thought I had misheard her, and stared at Connie for a couple of seconds, without saying anything. Jackie shot a look at me, and then back to her. I might have asked her to repeat herself, but I don't remember in my confusion.

"I'm not her sister," Connie said, reiterating the information as much for our benefit as for her own, as if she were testing what the words sounded like out loud. "I'm her mother. I'm Joan's mother. I had her when I was 15. I didn't want to give her up, but I couldn't raise her myself either, and my parents didn't want anyone to know I was pregnant. So I moved away from home for a few months, and had her, and when I came back we all just pretended my mother had another baby. Joan's grandmother. Joan was raised by her grandparents. And me."

On the wall close to the ceiling hung a large clock with black hands, numerals, and the manufacturer's name, *Seth Thomas*, prominent on its white face. The clock ticked away as we sat in silence. I wondered what other secrets had been disclosed in this room that Mr. Thomas was privy to.

"Does Joan know?" I asked.

Connie shook her head. "She doesn't. And I'd prefer she not find out. At least, not this way. Can't you just start looking in the Be The Match program?"

The cruelty of genetic randomness is that in some cases, it isn't so random, and uncovers truths that we didn't anticipate when we test siblings to see if one could be a bone marrow donor. More commonly, this involves paternal discrepancy.

One report focusing on paternal discrepancy—when a child is identified as being biologically fathered by someone other than the man who believes he is the father—identified 17 studies published between 1950 and 2004. Rates ranged between 0.8 percent and 30 percent, with a median rate of 3.7 percent. Older studies relied on blood type compatibility, whereas more contemporary ones applied DNA testing, similar to what would be used to assess whether or not one person is an HLA—and thus a bone marrow transplant—match for another.[18] Higher rates occurred in studies that included participants who were disputing paternity, as might be expected.

Rates of misattributed paternity (another catch-phrase for paternal discrepancy) among living related donors for bone marrow and solid organ transplantation ranges from 1 to 10 percent. Another study that examined the association between genetic signatures on the Y chromosome and surname in the United Kingdom found rates of non-paternity to be even lower, at approximately 1 in 25, or 4 percent.[19]

My conclusion from the sparse research on this topic is that rates of paternal discrepancy are low, but real, and are likely to be revealed more frequently as the rates of bone marrow transplantation increase.

What is our moral obligation, though, to both patients and donors, with respect to disclosing it?

A survey of 102 potential kidney transplant recipients, donors, and healthcare providers asked this very question.[20] Among 35 potential recipients, 60 percent wanted this information disclosed. Half of donors agreed, whereas only 43 percent of providers were willing to disclose paternal discrepancy. The providers' reluctance to disclose biologic paternity (relative to the percentage recipients and donors) stems from a number of factors.

First, even genetic testing can be wrong, and nobody would want to introduce such filial and marital havoc into a family without being absolutely sure of the results. This would follow principles of beneficence (to do good for the patient) and non-maleficence (to do no harm).[21]

Second, to whom does a physician or nurse have a primary obligation? His or her patient with leukemia, or the "patient" who is providing a blood sample to assess HLA compatibility? Turns out, both.[22]

I have an ethical and moral responsibility to maintain the confidentiality of my patients. A number of times, a well-meaning child has pulled me aside or requested to speak with me separately, without my patient present, to ask the question:

"How's Mom really doing?"

It's the same question I would want to ask my mother's physician if she had a serious illness. It's actually what I expected Connie to ask when she accompanied us to the conference room.

"What has she told you is going on?" I'll often reply. And most times, the child will then reflect back to me precisely what has transpired with my patient's health. But if not, I have to ask my patient's permission to discuss her health with any family member.

"Don't talk to him," one patient instructed me, referring to a physician brother who had called my office to review my patient's leukemia. "He's crazy and I don't want him involved in my healthcare."

I never would have guessed if I hadn't asked.

I also can't ethically disclose information I have learned about one patient to another—even when they are siblings, and even when one's chance of receiving a potentially curative bone marrow transplant depends on the other. This is referred to as the principlist approach to respecting autonomy: that patients (in this case, the patient supplying blood to assess if he or she could be a bone marrow donor) should have autonomy to make informed decisions based on information communicated by the healthcare provider, and that autonomy implies that a patient has the right to informed consent, confidentiality, and to control that information in maintaining privacy. Connie deliberately told us "I'd prefer she not find out."

Counter to this, genetics groups have recommended that incidental findings (in this case, the incidental finding of paternal or maternal discrepancy) noted on genetic screening tests should be reported to patients. Some have even advocated that the potential for such discrepancies be included in informed consent for HLA testing.

To deal with this and other potential conflicts between the rights of the donor and of the recipient, many bone marrow transplant groups assign different doctors, nurses, and even social workers to the donor from those who are assisting the recipient. This also mitigates the issue of *coercion*, where a donor may feel pressured by family members to undergo a procedure, with its attendant risks, that he or she really doesn't want to endure. Members of teams will report HLA testing results back to the potential donor, and ask permission if those results can be communicated to the potential recipient.[23] If paternal or maternal discrepancy arises, the teams simply disclose that the potential donor "was not a match."

"We'll start looking in the Be The Match registry for Joan. And we won't tell Joan what you just told us," I reassured Connie.

"We'll just say that you aren't a match for her. Which is true," Jackie added.

"Thank you," Connie said, resting her hands on the wood conference table. "To think, all these years of her not knowing. And that a bone marrow transplant, of all things, would have revealed it." She shook her head again. "Of all things."

7

A Life Extinguished, a Life Awakened

*. . . My father had dignity. At the
end of his life his life began
to wake in me.*

—Sharon Olds, "His Stillness," 1992

How strange, hearing the disconsolate cry of a newborn in a cancer center.

These monotonous white hallways—punctuated by honey-colored doors, sterile foaming cans, and subtle plastic "flags" by the door frames that indicate what room would be attended to by which doctor—conveyed professionalism, competence, cleanliness. The gray carpeting acted like a damper when important conversations occurring on the other side of the doors spilled out to the corridor: hushed tones, bursts of laughter, muffled relief, muted despair . . . but almost never the full-throated release of an infant demanding to be fed, NOW!

This kid had a set of lungs on him. Not wanting to add to the chaos, I waited until it sounded like Joseph Jr's needs were being met before I knocked on Sarah Badway's door and entered the room.

Sarah was sitting in the chair near the desk wearing black yoga pants and a purple top. She was cradling the baby, who was wrapped like a burrito in a white blanket with tiny gray elephants on it. A shock of black hair peeked out from a blue hat. He sucked away from a bottle of formula, all business, eyes half closed.

"It's about time you dropped by to meet Joey," Sarah scolded me. "Didn't you hear him call for you?"

"Honestly, I think habitants of remote regions of the Amazon basin heard him call for me." Sarah laughed. Her eyes looked tired. "He's a really handsome guy."

"Yeah, I think I'll keep him," she said, fussing with his hair.

"He sleeping okay?" I asked.

"Not bad. Goes to bed at 11 at night, wakes up at 4 for another bottle, then again at 7. I'll tell you, he sleeps better than the others did. I think it's the formula."

I had advised Sarah to avoid breastfeeding while taking the imatinib for her CML, as studies have shown that, in women taking the drug, amounts of it can be found in breast milk.[1] We didn't need Joey to receive the chemotherapy unnecessarily. His blood counts, checked by his pediatrician, were normal—there had been no vertical transmission of Sarah's leukemia.

"And how are you doing?"

"Better," she said, looking up from the baby to me. "I'm better. I won't lie to you, there are times when I'm dealing with him or with the others and I forget to take the medicine, but I remember it later on. I don't think I've missed a day," she reassured me.

"I could tell. Your blood counts look good. And the Philadelphia chromosome is almost gone."

We continue to assess the *BCR-ABL* genetic translocation of the Philadelphia chromosome every three months for the first couple of years of therapy, ensuring that the genetic abnormality exists in fewer and fewer cells over time. It's measured with a lab test called polymerase chain reaction, or PCR.

Invented in 1983 by Kary Mullis, PhD, who at the time was working for the Cetus Corporation in Northern California, PCR revolutionized the field of genetics and made possible many of the discoveries of genetic abnormalities found in cancer.[2]

On a drive through the mountains to a weekend cabin in Mendocino, inspiration hit Mullis for a better way to detect tiny genetic changes housed in the comparatively large chromosomes. He won the Nobel Prize in Chemistry a decade later for his work. Like so many brilliant scientific discoveries, it now seems relatively straightforward: Think of the gene sequence as the "words" that form the "books" of chromosomes. When we know the gene sequence that provides the instructions to make a protein (such as the tyrosine kinase in CML), a complementary gene sequence can be "zippered" to the original. With PCR, that zipper can be copied, and copied, and copied until you have thousands to millions more copies than you started with, allowing the abnormality to be detected, whereas before it may have been hidden within the thousands of genes on a single chromosome—a single misprinted word within a book. Using this approach, PCR can detect even one cell with the *BCR-ABL* translocation out of 50,000 cells or more.

Luckily, the *BCR-ABL* translocation can be assessed using a routine blood draw with about the same accuracy as a bone marrow test. At diagnosis, about 90 percent of Sarah's cells contained the *BCR-ABL* mutation. Three months later, that number was less than 10 percent of cells containing the mutation. At six months, it was at about 1 percent. Our goal was to get it to less than 0.1 percent.

Why so low? In the study that randomized more than 1,100 people with CML to receive either imatinib or what had been the standard therapy of interferon and cytarabine, in which 95 percent of patients treated with imatinib had normalization of their blood counts, 408 of the 553 people receiving imatinib had chromosomes that went back to normal—no longer showing the Philadelphia chromosome abnormality. Compare that to only 47 of the 553 people who received interferon and cytarabine. And 57 percent of those treated with imatinib who achieved this "chromosome remission" also had a 1,000-fold decrease in the *BCR-ABL* mutation that could be measured by PCR one year after starting their imatinib—thus reaching a level of less than 0.1 percent of cells with the mutation, our goal for Sarah.[3]

And none of the people in this 57 percent club had CML that worsened in the subsequent year of follow-up.

Sarah was on the right track with the timing of her falling *BCR-ABL* percentages, too. Another study of almost 300 people with CML treated with imatinib showed that those whose *BCR-ABL* levels were less than 10 percent at the three-month time point, like Sarah, were significantly more likely to be alive eight years later—with a 93 percent survival rate, compared to only 57 percent for those whose levels were greater than 10 percent.[4]

Imatinib is called a "tyrosine kinase inhibitor"—it blocks the abnormal CML protein (tyrosine kinase) produced by the Philadelphia chromosome that is stuck in an "on" position, which causes the cells to grow uncontrollably.

When Sarah was first diagnosed with CML, Rachel had asked about other more potent tyrosine kinase inhibitors—the "sons" and "daughters" of imatinib, called dasatinib and nilotinib. Two studies published in 2010 that enrolled almost 1,400 patients showed that the new drugs enabled significantly more CML patients—over 60 percent more—to achieve that magical *BCR-ABL* level of less than 0.1 percent. And they got to this milestone faster.[5]

Newer generation tyrosine kinase inhibitors—the grandchildren and great-grandchildren of imatinib—bosutinib and ponatanib—seem to work *even* better, albeit with different side effects to worry about.

So now that Sarah was no longer pregnant, the question remained as to whether I should recommend changing her treatment to one of these newer drugs. Well, with five-year follow-up of the "sons" and "daughters" trials, published in 2016, survival was similar for those treated with imatinib or with a son or daughter drug.[6] Since she was tolerating the medicine, taking it regularly, and achieving her milestones, why mess with success?

We had discussed whether to switch drugs just prior to Joey's birth. But despite her early missteps with taking the imatinib, Sarah had become almost protective of the drug, and didn't want to abandon it. She set phone alarms to remember to take her pill daily, and even left her amber pill bottle out on a shelf by her bathroom sink as a visual cue. She was proud of her new zealotry around medication compliance. She'd been bragging about it to me a few months earlier, around the time she was about to give birth to Joey.

"Go ahead, ask your question," she had challenged me when I saw her.

"Have you had any alcoholic beverages recently?" I asked.

Sarah looked at me like I was four kinds of idiot and gestured to her shirt. It was black with white lettering that read "SOBER . . . UNTIL MARCH." I laughed, though not without some hesitation given her past wild days. My favorite of her pregnancy shirts showed a computer's spinning wheel on her belly with the message "LOADING . . ." underneath.

"How have you been doing with taking your pills?" I obliged.

"100 percent perfect!" She was almost shouting. "No misses, all net!"

I congratulated her effusively, and she beamed. "When's the big day?"

"I scheduled the C-section for next Thursday," Sarah said. "Hey, and about that. A couple of my girlfriends asked if I was going to save the cord blood. Waddaya think?"

"Why are you considering it?" I asked.

She shrugged her shoulders a bit. "I dunno. Maybe for him, in case he gets cancer. Maybe for me if I ever need it."

Banking cord blood in case a bone marrow transplant is needed in the future is appealing on so many levels. The umbilical cord attaching the developing fetus to its mother's placenta is rich in those juicy bone marrow stem cells that are so effective at making the blood components. Coming from an infant at the time of birth, they should be uncorrupted by cancer. Cord blood is also easy to collect: At the time of delivery, after the cord is cut, the remaining blood in that cord is milked out into a collection bag. That bag is then kept in a freezer until the time comes, if ever, when it is needed and can be infused as a transplant.

The cost for this, using commercial cord blood banking companies, can be substantial. Upfront charges with what's called an enrollment fee can range from $1,500 to $3,500. On top of that, a yearly storage fee is assessed, with the total amount for 18 to 20 years of storage cresting $5,000 in some cases.[7] Brochures for these companies line Plexiglas display cases in obstetrics offices, with pamphlets exhorting nervous, expectant parents to protect their baby from the medical evils that lie ahead. What better source for a transplant than a child's own, pure stem cells, harvested at a time years before that child ever developed cancer? Is the cost and effort worth it for the risk that a child may one day develop a cancer and need a future transplant?

There are two ways of answering this question. First, what is the likelihood of a child developing a cancer, and then needing a transplant to treat that cancer?

A study conducted by the Center for International Blood and Marrow Transplant Research attempted to figure this out.[8] They first identified the cancers for which transplantation could potentially be needed. For people aged 0 to 19 years (the length of time a cord blood would be kept banked) leukemia was the most common, followed by lymphoma, neuroblastoma, brain tumors, and sarcomas. Cancer in children and adolescents are rare—all told, the incidence rate in the United States for all of these cancers combined was about 12 per 100,000 children per year. It's horrible if it's your child who develops cancer, but pediatric cancer is still an uncommon event.

The next conclusion is based on the likelihood that these cancers would not be eradicated by chemotherapy and/or radiation therapy and would require an allogeneic transplant—and the assumption that everyone could identify a sibling or "brother from another mother" transplant and was healthy enough to undergo a transplant. The authors estimated that the incidence rate of transplant for children and adolescents was a little over 2 per 100,000 per year in the United States during their first two decades of life. Analyzed another way, the probability a child will need a transplant by the time he or she reaches age 20 is 0.04 percent.

The lifetime chance of getting struck by lightning is similar, at about 1 in 3,000, or 0.033 percent.[9]

Would you pay thousands of dollars for a medication right now, in the event that sometime in your life you may be struck by lightning, and that medication may help you survive the lightning strike?

Seems excessive to me.

A second way of determining the value of cord blood banking in case a child develops cancer is to consider whether that cord blood is really as pure as we think.

The most common childhood cancer through age 19 is leukemia, with an annual incidence rate of 4.7 per 100,000 children in the United States.[10] Could it be possible that the leukemia was present at some small level even at birth, years before the child was diagnosed with leukemia?

One approach to studying this would be to screen every newborn for leukemia. Given the incidence rate of childhood leukemia, this would mean subjecting over 21,000 babies to a blood test for every case of future leukemia identified. It's difficult to justify that type of monumental screening effort to answer a research question about the origins of leukemia. A more reasonable approach would be to identify children who have leukemia, and try to determine whether they had it when they were born.

But how to go about obtaining a blood sample from a birth that occurred years earlier? A group of clever scientists from the United Kingdom and Germany thought the answer might be found in Guthrie cards.[11]

Robert Guthrie was a microbiologist working at the Roswell Park Cancer Institute in Buffalo, New York, in the 1950s when his niece was diagnosed with phenylketonuria (PKU), an inherited deficiency in the enzyme necessary to metabolize the amino acid phenylalanine. If caught early enough, an infant's diet can be modified so that the effects of the deficiency are minimized. If not, the condition can lead to developmental defects and mental retardation. Guthrie's niece was not so lucky. This, and having a child of his own with cognitive delays, motivated Guthrie to devote his career to detecting preventable childhood diseases. He developed a test for PKU that could be performed when a drop of blood from a finger prick or heel stick was applied to filter paper on a card. It was successfully piloted in Newark in 1960, and by 1963, 400,000 infants had been tested in 29 states. Testing spread around the country, and across the pond.[12]

And hospital laboratories kept those Guthrie cards for years after a child was born.

The scientists found three children with acute lymphocytic leukemia (more common in children than AML, whereas the opposite is true in adults) who had the same chromosome mutation associated with their leukemias—a translocation of chromosomes 4 and 11. After obtaining permission from the parents of these children, the scientists then searched laboratory repositories to find the Guthrie cards stored there from when the children were born. They used a PCR-specific lab test for this translocation on the dried blood still remaining on the children's Guthrie cards, and were able to detect the chromosome abnormality for all three children—from a blood drop obtained months or years before the leukemia was diagnosed. In another, similar study, the same group of scientists was able to detect chromosome evidence of leukemia in 9 of the 12 Guthrie cards obtained from children who diagnosed with leukemia between two and five years later.[13]

The leukemia was there all along, even prior to birth in these children, waiting years in some cases to rear its ugly head. And if the leukemia was measurable on a genetic level in their blood, it was almost certainly present in their cord blood. Banking cord blood from these children would have preserved those juicy, healthy stem cells, but also probably cells already corrupted by genetic abnormalities that would lead to leukemia—again, if the cells were reinfused into a child as a transplant years later.

Getting back to the question: Is the cost and effort of banking cord blood worth it for the risk that a child may one day develop a cancer and need a future transplant?

I didn't think so when my three children were born. But I did have their cord blood collected and I donated it to be stored for use through the Be The Match program, in case a complete stranger needed it someday. Maybe my children would be the brothers from another mother, or sister from another mister—me being the mister!

In Sarah's case, banking cord blood was probably overkill. Given her chances of doing well on imatinib or a similar drug, she was unlikely to ever need a transplant. If she did, her best options would be a sibling or a matched, unrelated donor, not one of her own children. And even if that didn't work out for her, and she did need a transplant from a child, she has other, older children to choose from who could donate marrow to her at the time she needs it, avoiding all of those cord blood storage enrollment and storage costs.

In any case, there was still the possibility that Joey's cord blood was contaminated with her leukemia. For all of these reasons, Sarah decided against saving Joey's cord blood.

As Joey sucked out the dregs of formula, the bottle dropped gently from his lips, and his head lolled back as he fell asleep. Sarah expertly took the bottle away, and with one hand capped it and placed it in the brown diaper bag sitting on the chair beside her. The bag had the same gray elephant design on it as Joey's blanket.

"Any side effects to the chemo? Nausea? Leg cramps?" I asked softly, trying not to wake the baby.

"All good," Sarah answered, in her regular voice. "And doc, no need to whisper. If this kid doesn't learn to nap with chaos, he'll never get any sleep in my house."

I laughed as Sarah got up from her chair to put Joey in his car seat, and then sat on the examination table. I checked her from head to toes, asking permission before feeling her neck for lymph nodes. As a medical student, I once examined a women's neck without asking permission, and she told me it felt as if I were choking her. I later learned that she had been the victim of domestic violence, during which her partner throttled her. I hadn't appreciated the intimacy of the dance of the physical exam before that. Because of her feedback, I've been careful in asking permission to perform exams my entire career.

When I finished, I went to the sink to wash my hands. Sarah gathered her jacket, the diaper bag, and finally the car seat with Joey in it, dead to the world. She swung it gently, rocking him, without even realizing it.

"So, I'm fine for another three months?" she asked. I nodded. "Any chance I can stop taking the chemo?" She smiled at me, acknowledging that the question was a long shot.

It wasn't as absurd as she might have thought. A couple of studies conducted in Australia and Europe asked just this question: Can imatinib be stopped in people whose *BCR-ABL* was not detectable using the PCR test?[14]

In the Australian study, 40 CML patients whose PCR for the *BCR-ABL* abnormality was negative for two straight years stopped taking their imatinib. With a median follow-up of 3.5 years, 18 of those patients remained in remission and off their drug, without evidence that the CML had returned. All of the 22 patients whose CML returned restarted their imatinib, and all regained their remission. Unfortunately, not all were able to have the same continuous period of negative PCR that first made them eligible for the study.

In a study from France, 100 CML patients whose PCR was negative for two years also stopped their imatinib. With a median 17 months of follow-up, 54 patients had *BCR-ABL* that returned—a similar percentage as in the Australian study. In a follow-up study conducted at a number of institutions across Europe, more than 750 CML patients with a negative PCR for one year stopped imatinib or other tyrosine kinase inhibitors and were followed for a median of 27 months. About half of these patients (371) had *BCR-ABL* that returned, and about 300 regained their *BCR-ABL* negative status after restarting their drug.[15]

A "glass half full" sort of person might conclude that all those with CML who reach that benchmark of persistent, negative PCR should have a chance at stopping their chemotherapy. A "glass half empty" person might instead think it nuts to stop what is arguably the most effective chemotherapy ever developed, when half of those people had a relapse of their leukemia.

What happened to the people enrolled in the European studies whose leukemia returned? They were restarted on their imatinib, or a son or daughter of imatinib, and most reentered a leukemia-free state. But not all, and it still isn't known for how long they were able to recapture their remissions.

The point was moot for Sarah, as we could still detect her *BCR-ABL*.

"Not anytime soon. But there may come a point when we can discuss it. Keep up the good work with taking the medicine," I said to her, turning from the sink to face her. "Hey, and try to stay out of trouble," I joked.

"Doc, I got a birthday coming up, and me and my friends are going to rent one of those vans with a driver who can take us around to different bars, to celebrate." She opened the room's door and walked out. "But don't you worry, I won't forget to take the pill!"

Sarah walked away from me down the carpeted hallway, still swinging Joey's car seat, before I could say anything. She was returning to family, friends, and her responsibilities outside her doctor's appointments.

I enter my patients' lives *in medias res*, as an interloper conscripted to battle disease, and I do my damnedest to rid them of the malignant golem. But they often come to me with a lifetime of destructive behaviors, and with other medical conditions that preceded the leukemia. And much as I try, I don't always have the same impact on those other problems.

Later that morning, I checked David's vital signs scribbled on the paper hanging by his examination room. His blood pressure was "skimming trees" at 98/58, and his heart was clicking away at a rate of 112 beats per minute. He had a low-grade fever at 99 and change.

I knocked on the door and entered. Just as I was about to shut it, I felt a push on it from behind as Rachel squeezed in behind me.

"Sorry!" she whispered as she shut the door behind us.

David sat in a wheelchair by the desk. The room was packed, just as it had been the day we broke the news to the whole Sweeney family that his leukemia had never gone away. He was wearing a Cleveland Indians cap and sweatshirt. So was Betty. Opening day for the team was just a week away, and a bunch of my patients were similarly outfitted, as if through this act of sartorial intimidation they could bully winter into submission and clear the way for spring to finally arrive in Cleveland. The weather in northeast Ohio has a reputation for shrugging its shoulders at these vainglorious attempts; on opening day in April 2007, it dumped enough snow to cancel a game against the Seattle Mariners one pitch before becoming official. In protest one fan ran onto the field, threw himself on the ground, and made a snow angel in right-center field. With typical Cleveland self-effacing humor, the stadium's PA system played Bing Crosby's "White Christmas" during a second-inning delay.[16]

The cap looked two sizes too big for David's head. He had lost weight, and as his tissue had wasted, the bones around his eyes became more prominent. He still had some of his tan from a recent trip he took with his family, and the darker color belied the degree of anemia he had. Betty looked tired, more resigned, though, than sad. Susan had taken her usual spot on the exam table, and for reasons I'll never be able to explain regarding the haphazard migration patterns of chairs in the hospital, we were blessed with an additional chair for Eric. So he sat across from his parents and along with Susan greeted us with a smile. As I moved to sit next to David, I saw Rachel mouth to Eric "How are you?" and watched him give her the thumbs-up sign.

David had decided to try the pill that targets the *IDH2* mutation found in his leukemia. It took a couple of weeks to clear some insurance hurdles to guarantee the pills would be mostly covered (the drug was priced even higher than other oral chemotherapy for leukemia, at the gasp-inducing cost of $30,000 per month). When he started the treatment, he again experienced nausea like he had in the hospital—not quite as bad, but not good, either. Betty, Susan, and Eric alternately drove him to clinic twice weekly for transfusions. At the same time we could monitor his labs and his symptoms for the differentiation syndrome. Sure enough, three weeks into his treatment, he came to clinic short of breath with a fever and rising white blood cell count.

We admitted him to the hospital and started him on steroids, just as we had for Joan when she had the differentiation syndrome while taking her ATRA. Whether it was feeling sick again, or the toll that making multiple trips into Cleveland had taken on him, or the reminder of what it felt like to be hospitalized so soon after he had returned to living at home, David declared enough was enough.

"I can't do this anymore," he had said to us while lying in his hospital bed. Clear plastic tubes wrapped over his ears to supply oxygen to his nose. Only Betty was with him that day. "This is not a life."

"You can stop anytime you want. You're the boss," I had reminded him. "But what if we can get you feeling better with the steroids, and figure out a better regimen to get rid of the nausea?"

He shook his head, and then started to cry. "I can't, I just can't." He covered his face with his hands for a few seconds, quietly sobbing, his shoulders shaking, as Betty moved from her chair to his bed and sat beside him. She hugged him, holding his head and stroking his hair, and soothed him, saying "it's okay" over and over.

"I'm sorry," he said to her. "I don't want to let you and the kids down. I'm sorry."

She shook her head and started crying herself. "You did everything, honey. You've been so brave. It's okay to stop. We can't ask anything more of you."

I sat quietly in the chair by his bed as they comforted each other, watching this husband and wife soothe each other with words and touches in a way that only people who have been together for decades know.

"David?" I said gently, waiting for him to look up. "Let's stop the pills. It's the right decision."

He lifted his hands from his face and nodded. "Thank you," he answered, barely audible.

Later that day I returned to his room to ask how far he wanted to go in stopping his treatments, and how he wanted to live the rest of his life.

"What are my options?" David was sitting up in bed, having regained his composure from earlier in the day, and was back to his pragmatic self.

"We can be as aggressive as you'd like. Some people with leukemia who don't want the chemo any more still do want to receive blood and platelet transfusions, and even antibiotics if they have an infection. Others don't want any contact with a clinic or hospital, and choose more of a hospice approach. You'd remain at home, and a nurse would visit you there, and even help provide you with medications to allow you to be comfortable and to live your life as fully as possible."

"Can't he have both?" Betty asked. "Transfusions and hospice?"

It was a great question. Hospice presents unique challenges in an end-of-life leukemia population, not the least of which centers on leukemia patients needing blood and platelet transfusions to survive. Why would simple blood and platelet transfusions be so hard?

Transfusions of blood products can only be performed in a clinic or hospital, making the logistics of transfusions challenging for a person who is on hospice and homebound.[17] Family members of a few of my end-stage leukemia patients have told me it may take them two hours to help my patient wash, dress, and transfer to a car so that person can make it to clinic for a transfusion. At a certain point, it just gets to be too much effort for everyone.

The cost of regular transfusions also exceeds the per diem payment that hospice agencies receive to care for an individual. Many such agencies will not willingly allow a treatment that could put them out of business, harsh as that sounds. A few more enlightened agencies will, though.

Some even argue that blood and platelet transfusions are considered "heroic" therapies, and thus are antithetical to the philosophy of some hospice groups that avoid aggressive treatment of a disease and focus instead on symptom control. Yet a study of more than 100 cancer patients receiving palliative care showed that those receiving red blood cell transfusions had improvement in symptoms of fatigue, breathlessness, weakness, or dizziness.

Whatever the reason, one survey of almost 350 US hematologist/oncologists found that this inability for patients to receive transfusions was a barrier to hospice referral for 62 percent of respondents. From a patient perspective, there are analyses using data from Medicare and from the Surveillance Epidemiology and End Results (SEER) program of the Centers for Disease Control and the National Cancer Institute—one including almost 7,000 patients, the other 21,000: Those with leukemia or myelodysplastic syndrome (the bone marrow condition we suspected of preceding David's leukemia) who were dependent on blood transfusions were 31 percent less likely to use hospice.[18] For those who did use hospice, they spent a significantly shorter amount of time in hospice (at a median of 6 versus 11 days), and a separate analysis showed that they were significantly more likely to die in the hospital, rather than at home.

"I still want the transfusions," David said. "I can't go long without getting blood and platelets, right?" He had been receiving a transfusion of each every week or two. I nodded in response. "Well, then let's just continue those and hold off on hospice for now."

"How soon can he get out of the hospital?" Betty asked, having returned to her chair.

"A day or two, let's make sure this differentiation syndrome has gotten better and that David doesn't have an infection," I answered.

"Good. We decided that we want to go on a trip down to Florida, to the Gulf Coast. We go down there every year around this time. Is that possible?" David asked.

I nodded again. "We'll have to work it around your transfusions, and I'd like to find a hospital near where you're heading, so that if you get sick you'll know where to go. But if that's what's important to you, we'll make it happen."

David seemed satisfied, and lay back on his pillows. "I want to spend the week with my family, sitting in a chair staring at the ocean, just thinking about where we all came from."

Too many leukemia patients at the end of life spend their time in clinic or in the hospital. One study of 330 people with AML diagnosed between 2005 and 2011 found that, once diagnosed with leukemia, patients were hospitalized four times on average. Those who died spent over 28 percent of their lives from the moment of diagnosis in the hospital and almost 14 percent in clinic. Within 30 days of death, 85 percent were hospitalized, 45 percent had received some type of chemotherapy, and 61 percent died in the hospital.[19]

In addition to the operational and economic hurdles in engaging hospice, and the reluctance of doctors and nurses to stop therapy once it's been started, a more subtle explanation for high hospitalization and treatment rates at the end of a leukemia patient's life is that people's goals change, sometimes suddenly. It often takes a sentinel event like a side effect to chemotherapy, or yet another hospitalization, for a person to realize, "I can't do this anymore." When the treatment brakes are applied for a fast-growing cancer like leukemia, it may not take long, even less than 30 days, for a person to die from the disease.

Two months later, David sat in clinic wearing his Indians gear. Fortunately, he hadn't gotten any infections since his hospitalization, and the frequency with which he needed transfusions had been pretty stable, until recently. He now needed blood or platelets two or three times each week.

Rachel and I saw him often, sometimes alone with Betty, sometimes with her and Susan, and occasionally with Eric. Rachel got to know Eric better, and even apologized for how she had reacted to him. Water under the bridge, now.

When David made his decision about not receiving any more chemotherapy, Susan and Eric supported him. Maybe it took tincture of time, maybe it was seeing what he had endured at the hands of his disease and the chemotherapy. Maybe it took staring at the Gulf of Mexico, thinking about where we all came from.

"It's getting to be a lot, coming in here all the time," David said, his voice not as resonant as it once was. "On me and on all of them."

Susan rolled her eyes. "Daddy, it's no trouble for us at all. It's nice we get some time alone with you."

David smiled at how she soft-pedaled the disruption to her life, to all of their lives. They had raised her well. He continued. "I'm thinking it might be time we get that hospice involved and stop these transfusions."

"We've worn out our welcome, have we?" I asked.

He smiled again, wanly. "Besides, I don't want to miss opening day next week because I'm sitting in one of your infusion chairs."

"That would be my choice, too," I told him.

Could David make it long enough to see opening day? I've long been convinced that, at least to some extent, and within the boundaries imposed by the aggressiveness of their cancers, my patients die only when they're good and ready to. For many, that time occurs after they have achieved a specific goal. Perhaps it's the birth of a grandchild, or that grandchild's college graduation. Maybe it's seeing the long-lost sibling a patient has been feuding with for years. Parents always wait to say goodbye to their children: I have seen patients, even those moribund and comatose, linger for days until a daughter or son from overseas arrives.

One patient, a man in his late 60s who had multiple cancers, told me his goal was to walk his granddaughter down the aisle at her wedding.[20] He and his wife had raised her while their daughter, who had gotten pregnant in her teens and then became addicted to drugs, struggled to get her life back in order.

After surviving colon cancer years earlier, he developed lung cancer. Prior to treating that cancer, the lung cancer specialist referred him to me when he noticed the patient had abnormal blood counts. A bone marrow biopsy revealed both acute leukemia and *another* bone marrow cancer, multiple myeloma.

Three cancers at the same time, four in total, but you'd never know it from his attitude.

Determined, positive, and uncompromising: none of these cancers would keep him from that wedding. The chemotherapy knocked his blood counts down, but didn't do much to kill the leukemia. The lung cancer spread to his brain, leaving him partially paralyzed. We treated that well enough, with steroids, so he could walk again.

"You should have heard the gasp from everyone in the church when he came through those doors with our granddaughter," his wife told me. "No one thought he would be there."

But I did.

I saw him one last time after the wedding. He wore a sweatshirt with a photo transfer of him and his granddaughter walking down the aisle. The caption read "Mission Accomplished."

This kind of "will-to-live-until" phenomenon has even been studied. Investigators from Ohio State University explored whether people with cancer die soon after they achieve a milestone, which for the study was defined as a birthday, Thanksgiving, or Christmas.[21] They examined death certificates from over 300,000 people who died with cancer in Ohio during an 11-year period, from 1989 to 2000. It was a negative study, though; people with cancer were no more likely to die after these events than before.

The authors concluded: "Analysis of thousands of cancer deaths shows no pattern to support the concept that 'death takes a holiday.' We find no evidence that cancer patients are able to postpone their death to survive Christmas, Thanksgiving, or their own birthdays."

But I've always felt the study focused on the wrong "milestone." I haven't looked forward to a birthday for decades, and when I did it was only at seminal transitions: from 15 to 16, when I could finally drive my mom's Toyota Tercel, and 20 to 21, when I could hold my head high as I walked into a bar in my home state of Rhode Island using my real driver's license, not the one claiming I was from Lumberton, New Jersey. Holidays are a mixed blessing for even the most hale and hearty of us, particularly if they involve travel with young children hopped up on sugar, and an unwelcome break from routine.

The other people I've witnessed who seem to have some say in when a dramatic, health-related life event will occur are pregnant women. I can't count the number of times during my wife's pregnancies when someone commented that she would go into labor only after she'd "finished nesting"—that is, preparing for the birth and completing other tasks she needed to accomplish before going on maternity leave. Put these two together—a person on the cusp of dying, and a pregnant woman at term—and we have the makings of a serious stalemate.

A few years back, I cared for a woman who had end-stage cancer. She had slipped into a coma, but before doing so declared that she wanted to live long enough to see the birth of her first grandchild. Her 40-week-pregnant daughter, who was by her side daily in the hospital, declared that she would not leave her mother to go into labor, for fear that she wouldn't be present when her mother took her last breath.

We witnessed this standoff for almost two weeks, until the daughter's obstetrician felt it was too dangerous to let the pregnancy continue any longer. The daughter left, reluctantly, to have a Caesarian section, returned hours later with the baby in her arms, and her mother died later that night.

Coincidence?

I think I would live long enough for one of those impossible-to-measure-in-a-study family-life events.

Some people have such tight relationships with sports teams that those teams figure prominently in death plans. One famous Cleveland fan, Scott Entsminger, made a request in his *Columbus Dispatch* obituary that six members of the Browns football team serve as his pallbearers "so the Browns can let him down one last time."[22] It wasn't a complete surprise, then, for David, with his family all around him, to focus his death plans on the Cleveland Indians.

"Goodbye, and good luck, David. It's been really nice getting to know you." As I rose from the chair, I held out my hand to shake David's. He took hold of it, and my gaze, for a few final seconds. We both knew this would be the last time we would see each other. I hugged Betty and Susan, and Rachel hugged Eric goodbye.

He made it to see the Indians opener on TV, and died the following day. The Tribe even managed to win the game, in 10 innings.

"Are you ready for your new birthday, Joan?" asked Tina, her nurse.

Joan was lying in a bed in the bone marrow transplant unit, around the bend from where she had just spent another four weeks on the leukemia service. Fortunately, that round of chemotherapy had done the trick and knocked her back into a remission. Also fortunately, her transplant team had been able to identify five potential matches through the Be The Match database. They chose the youngest, a 32-year-old man who was living in Western Europe. A study of almost 1,300 acute leukemia patients in Europe undergoing transplant over a 10-year period found that patients over the age of 40 were significantly affected by increasing donor age, with a higher likelihood the leukemia would return and worsen overall survival if the donor were older than 40.[23] The European man happened to be available and willing to donate his marrow; eight weeks after her discharge from the leukemia service, Joan was ready to receive it with open arms.

Well, with an open marrow. Joan had been in the transplant unit for about a week receiving a "preparative regimen" of chemotherapy to wipe out any remaining leukemia cells and any normal stem cells populating her marrow. As a result, her platelets and white and red blood cells were in the toilet. Her donor's marrow would now rescue this wasteland by repopulating it, which would take three to four weeks. We would know this had happened because her blood counts would recover—with blood cells manufactured by her donor's marrow, hopefully.

"I've decided to name him Lars," Joan declared.

"Your donor?" her best friend Patty asked. She was sitting in a chair by Joan's bed, as was Connie.

Joan nodded. "I've also decided he's six-foot-four, with piercing blue eyes and a beautiful head of blond hair." She ran her hand distractedly over the peach fuzz of brown hair on her own head. "He's an independently wealthy businessman who likes to sail, travel to exotic places like Canton, Ohio, and cater to my every need."

"Another independently wealthy boyfriend? Jeez, Joan, you collect them like candy!" Patty teased her.

"Can you actually find out who he is?" Connie asked.

"Only after a year. I have to give permission, and he has to give permission, and then I'm allowed to contact him."

"Joanie, you sure you have the energy for a guy 16 years younger than you?" Patty asked.

"You're about to find out!" Tina said, as she lifted the bag of cells and hung it on Joan's IV pole. It looked smaller than Joan expected, for all of the effort it took to get those precious cells. Slightly bigger than a bag of blood, and a similar shade of red.

"You sure those are the right ones?" Joan asked Tina, only half joking.

"I checked them three times, together with Janey. So did the cell-processing lab. These are your cells."

"I looked at 'em also Joanie, you're good to go." Patty added.

Joan sighed. "Okay, okay, I trust you. Let 'er rip!"

Tina attached the tubing between the bag of cells and the long-term Hickman catheter inserted into one of the major veins in Joan's chest. The red liquid started flowing.[24]

"When should I start sucking on the mints?" Joan asked. A bowl of wintergreen Lifesavers, individually wrapped in clear plastic, sat on her bedside table.

"Yeah, what's up with those?" Patty asked.

"Now is good," Tina told Joan. "The bone marrow was frozen to transport it overseas. It was placed in a preservative called DMSO that can cause a strong taste of garlic or creamed corn in your mouth. The mints help make that more tolerable."

"My skin may even smell like garlic," Joan added.

"You better hope Lars isn't a vampire, Joanie!" Patty laughed.

They were quiet for a little while, watching the cells in the bag slowly deplete as they flowed into Joan.

"Oooh, I'm getting the taste now," Joan said, reaching for another mint. She looked up at what remained in the bag of cells as she unwrapped one of the Lifesavers and popped it into her mouth. "It's kind of anticlimactic after all this, isn't it?"

"I'm good with that," Tina said. "We don't like excitement around here."

They were quiet again, watching the bag. Then, a knock on the open door and I walked in. I had been watching and listening to them from the nurse's station, the ebb and flow of their conversation, the quiet looks they gave each other. Hope, support, anticipation, worry, hope, support. The cycle of cancer emotions.

"Happy birthday, Joan," I said, suspecting Tina had already wished her the same.

"I'm not sure I'm ready to switch over from being a Virgo to . . . what sign is it now? Aries?" Joan asked.

"Pisces," Connie said. "You're a Pisces now."

"I don't even like fish," Joan said miserably. We all laughed. "And what blood type will I be?"

"You should just be grateful Lars is such a good match," Patty said. She turned to me and clarified, "Joan named her donor."

"When Lars's bone marrow takes over, you'll go from being O positive to B positive," Tina reminded her.

"Be positive," Joan repeated. "I'll do my best."

"It doesn't take over immediately?" Patty asked.

"Nope. For a while, the two bone marrows, Joan's and her donor's, will coexist," I explained. "Actually, coexist seems almost too hospitable. A battle will ensue over land rights to the precious space in Joan's bones. The majority of the time, the healthy donor bone marrow wins, which usually takes a few weeks. But until then, we'll be able to see both sets of bone marrow cells hard at work—what we call a chimeric bone marrow."

"Chimeric?" Connie asked.

"From Greek mythology. The Chimera was an animal with a lion's head, a goat's body, and a serpent's tail. For a while, your bone marrow will be part you, and part Lars."

"Maybe I should have named my donor Aristotle," Joan mused. She shook her head. "I was sure Connie would be a match. Only 25 percent chance though, huh?"

Connie held a thin smile and looked down at her hands, which were kneaded in a tight ball in her lap. What must be going through her mind at that moment, I couldn't imagine. Maybe Connie wished she had never participated in the ruse of treating Joan as her sister. Easy to say now,

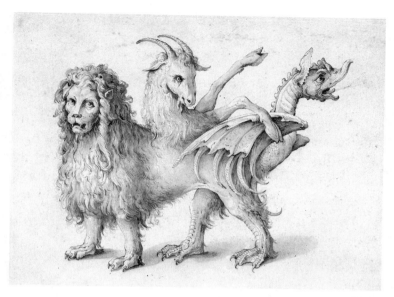

Figure 7.1
The Chimera from Greek mythology.

hard when you're a teenager almost 50 years ago whose parents may have declared it was this or adoption—or getting kicked out of the house. Maybe she should have told Joan the truth before the transplant. But Joan had enough to deal with then, with her leukemia returning, being admitted to the hospital for more chemotherapy, the very real threat of dying. One day, Connie promised herself. When Joan was better.

"Lars is a perfect match. About as good as a sibling." I had answered quickly, not wanting the awkwardness, of which only Connie and I were aware, to linger for too long.

"You called him my 'brother from another mother,'" Joan reminded me.

It wasn't the first time a patient came back at me with one of my quips. Years earlier, I cared for another nurse, this one in her late 20s, with acute lymphocytic leukemia. A fellow I was training, originally from Lebanon, followed her along with me. She had a wicked sense of humor, and our formal medical encounters often degenerated into silliness. At the end of the first year after her diagnosis, when she had completed six months of intensive chemotherapy and was receiving lower-dose chemo—what we called the maintenance phase of her treatment—she handed us each a piece of heavy stock paper.

"What's this?" I asked her.

"A top 10 list," she answered simply, waiting for us to review it.

I looked down and read the first few lines.

"He's sunshine. I'm a spotless mind."

"I have six months of fellowship left. If I pass."

"A lot of times in medicine we don't know why we do things. We just do them."

"You can't eat hummingbirds in this country."

I laughed, suddenly realizing what she had done. At the end of her visits with us, she had recorded some of the more outrageous comments we had made to her. The first occurred shortly after the Kate Winslet and Jim Carrey movie *Eternal Sunshine of the Spotless Mind* had been released in theaters. The last one derived from a tangent my fellow had once embarked upon of Lebanese delicacies.

At the time they were funny. Reading them in stark black ink with the crisp, white background, though, they were a bit jarring. It taught me how much the words we use in talking about leukemia matter, more than we may realize at the time. She presented us with a list every year, our annual ritual, until her leukemia recurred. She got too sick to record our comments, and the tone of our conversations reflected that, leaving little room for levity. She died by the time her third list would have been created.

"Do siblings who are perfect matches for each other look or act the same?" Patty asked.

I shook my head. "No way. From what I've seen, the sibling who's a match is usually the wild brother with the long beard who lives in the one-room shack in Montana writing his manifesto. The one everyone has always thought was adopted."

Joan laughed. "That definitely is not Connie."

Patty nodded as Joan continued smiling at the thought of her straight-and-narrow sister living off the grid.

"Once I break out of this joint, I'm basically under house arrest for a hundred days, right?" Joan asked.

"Yup. You will be so immuno-compromised as these bone marrow cells wage war on each other, and the new marrow starts to make new cells, that we want you to live within an hour of the hospital. That's in case you spike a fever or develop graft versus host disease, where the new immune system attacks some of your normal tissue." I explained, more for Patty and Connie's benefit, because Joan had already learned as much from her transplant team.

"I'll watch her like a hawk," Connie said, protectively. She would be Joan's caregiver during the hundred days.

"All done," Tina declared, as the final drops of cells flowed through the IV line. You feeling okay?" she asked Joan.

"I still have that garlic taste, but otherwise yeah, fine." Sometimes people can have an allergic reaction to the infusion, just as they might to a bag of blood or platelets. But for Joan, it had been smooth sailing.

Tina detached the bag and cleaned the medical detritus from the procedure off the bedside table.

"My services are clearly no longer needed here," I said, getting ready to leave. "Have a quiet day, Joan."

"You too, doc," Joan said. Connie mouthed "thank you" to me from across the room. Patty gave the thumbs-up sign.

As I walked out I ran into Rachel in the hallway.

"Did Joan get her cells?" she asked.

"All infused and accounted for."

"Any reaction?"

I shook my head. Rachel poked her head into the room, waved to Joan, and wished her a happy birthday.

"You ready to hear about this new admission in bed 4?" she asked me.

"Names, not numbers," I gently reminded Rachel, and took a fresh 3×5 card from the pocket of my white coat. The inexorable cycle of illness continued. "Go for it."

"Mr. Jensen is a 37-year-old man who was in his usual state of health until about three weeks ago, when he began to experience flu-like symptoms . . ."

Epilogue

Joan was discharged from the hospital 24 days later after her blood counts started to recover, which indicated that Lars's bone marrow had engrafted within her. She had bouts of graft versus host disease over the ensuing months, and a couple of fevers that landed her back in the hospital. One of those fevers—caused by respiratory syncytial virus, or RSV, the virus that leads to croup in children, but which can be deadly to a person with no immune system—landed her in the ICU again. But she remained in remission three years and counting following her transplant. Playing the odds, she was more likely cured than not.

She returned to work about a year after her diagnosis. The first time she scrubbed back into the OR for a case (another hernia repair!), a round of applause greeted her, led by the surgeon she had worked with for so long. He had visited her a few times during her multiple stays at the hotel Cleveland Clinic. She may even have seen his eyes tear up above his blue surgical mask.

Cure is a funny word within cancer circles. For people with leukemia, it is defined as having gone five years without the leukemia returning. But most oncologists I know, and patients too, avoid using the word with an almost religious or superstitious fervor.[1] A few times, earlier in my career, I told patients they were cured after we celebrated their five-year follow-up visit. Months later, a couple of them returned to my clinic with new laboratory abnormalities, and bone marrows that showed leukemia precursor diseases, such as myelodysplastic syndrome. Perhaps the chemotherapy we used to treat their leukemias knocked their bone marrows back to a primordial, pre-leukemia state that was now rearing its ugly head again. Perhaps the chemotherapy itself had caused the bone marrow changes. Regardless of the scenario, I became much more cautious in using the word.

I think we all fear that if we declare a person cured, we will be tempting the gods, and might accidently raise the malignant golem from its torpor. So instead, our focus is on phrases like "continued remission," or "durable remission." And we knock on a lot of particleboard tabletops for good luck when we use them.

The treatment of acute leukemia has become much more sophisticated, ranging from the use of new drugs that are "personalized" to attack the distinct genetic basis of the leukemia an individual has developed, to the incorporation of our new understanding of the genetic basis of leukemia so we can predict who would most likely benefit from a bone marrow transplant before the leukemia relapses.

The US Food and Drug Administration has just approved drugs like midostaurin and gilteritinib, which target a genetic abnormality called *FLT3*, which is present in about one-third of AML patients, because they extend people's lives.[2] Similarly, the drug David received briefly, enasidinib, and ivosidenib target the genetic mutations *IDH2* and *IDH1* (found in about 15 percent of people with AML) and in so doing induce responses in about one-third of patients whose AML has relapsed.[3] These drugs are also being incorporated into treatment after a bone marrow transplant, to prevent the leukemia from returning.

But what is available for the other 52 percent of AML patients who don't have a *FLT3* or *IDH* abnormality?

Other drugs in development are targeting additional genetic mutations. These mutations include *TP53*, which drives a leukemia that is exquisitely resilient to chemotherapy and portends particularly poor outcomes, as well as *SF3B1*, or a variety of other genetic mutations that affect a small percentage of leukemia patients and are similarly named with mixes of letters and numbers.[4]

My dad, a former newspaper reporter and no slouch in the "knows how to doggedly ask questions" department, once grilled me with a line of inquiries that boiled down to "Why can't researchers find a cure for cancer?"

Never mind cancer as a whole—leukemia itself is not one cancer, but dozens of cancers, each with its own distinct genetic fingerprint. Given the genetic complexity of leukemia, the future of therapeutic approaches will involve the need for many drugs, each of which targets a different genetic component of leukemia specific to just a small percentage of patients, and likely used in conjunction with standard chemotherapy.

Alternatively, there is immunotherapy, which takes advantage of a patient's own immune system to combat cancer. Being broadly similar in principle to the primary effect of bone marrow transplantation, it is being studied extensively in acute lymphocytic leukemia.[5] One approach involves chimeric antigen receptor (CAR) T-Cells, in which the immune system is deliberately exposed to a patient's particular leukemia outside the body to target that leukemia. The immune system portion targeting the leukemia is allowed to expand, and is reinfused into the body to attack the leukemia where it lives. Specific CAR T-Cells have been approved for lymphomas and for children, adolescents, and young adults with acute lymphocytic leukemia. Their response rates in these patient populations, many of whom had no other treatment options left, have been remarkable, even nearing 90 percent, with 50 percent of patients remaining in remission one year after they receive their immune cell infusion. Whether they work as well in myeloid cancers, such as acute myeloid leukemia, is being explored.

Sarah's *BCR-ABL* levels continued to decrease, crossing the magical Rubicon of being less than 0.1 percent. They never disappeared entirely, though, so stopping the imatinib was not in the cards. Years later, she started her own business and found time on top of that to join Joey's school's PTO. She rarely, if ever, missed a dose of the chemotherapy, and she managed to keep her drinking in check. Joey grew to be a healthy boy, his exposure to the imatinib in utero a non-issue. Although Sarah, still spirited as ever, blamed the drug for his being a "royal pain-in-the-ass."

Because we've seen so much success treating CML, given the effectiveness of imatinib and other tyrosine kinase inhibitor drugs, in some ways we leukemia caregivers and researchers have the luxury of focusing on more nuanced therapy questions: Can we stop treatment in patients whose PCR for the *BCR-ABL* mutation of the Philadelphia chromosome has gone negative? How negative is negative enough: A test that can detect 1 in 1,000 cells with the *BCR-ABL*, or 1 in 50,000? Can we reduce the dose of imatinib's children and grandchildren without losing efficacy? How can we help the minority of patients who don't fare well on the usual tyrosine kinase inhibitors?

When imatinib and its children or grandchildren don't work, it's usually because a person's CML has acquired an additional mutation that prevents the tyrosine kinase inhibitor drug from fitting neatly in the "pocket" of the tyrosine kinase protein that it is supposed to inhibit. A common mutation—and yes, its name comprises another series of letters and numbers—is *T315I*. Some grandchildren and even great-grandchildren of imatinib have been developed to help patients with just such a resistant CML. But with the improved efficacy comes additional side effects, such as a higher risk of forming blood clots, a risk increasingly detected as more and more CML patients, whose lives used to be measured in a handful of years, become decades-long survivors. Drug development in CML is focusing more on those rare patients for whom the approved tyrosine kinase inhibitors don't work, and in recognizing side effects in long-term survivors.[6]

David was buried in Ashtabula, in the same cemetery as his parents and grandparents were interred. More than a hundred people attended the service. Eric gave a moving eulogy on how hard it was to finally let his father go, and how his dad only slipped away after he and Susan gave him permission to do so.

I've heard palliative care and hospice nurses refer to the transition stage of death, similar to the transition stage of birth, usually the point at which a woman declares, "GET THIS BABY OUT!!!!" in no uncertain terms. The path to dying can be equally treacherous, equally painful. Having your children reassure you that you don't have to worry about them, that they will be okay without you, can make that journey more bearable.

At the unveiling of the gravestone, weeks later, Susan stuck a small Indians flag in the ground by his grave, along with a "We're #1!" Indians foam finger. His was not the only plot in the cemetery with those memorabilia.

Older adults with AML are probably the most challenging group of patients to treat, in large part because the biology and genetics of their cancers is even more complex than that in younger adults. Consequently, "one size fits all" treatment approaches are least likely to work, particularly as older patients tend not to have the "good risk" types of leukemia (as fraught with irony as that term is). Joan's acute promyelocytic leukemia is an example.

But what if we could identify which of these patients would benefit from more intensive therapy, and which from less intensive, outpatient therapy, at the time of their diagnosis? One approach to doing this lies in the power of computers to analyze pathologic, clinical, and genetic data using what's called "machine learning" or "artificial intelligence (AI)" programming.

AI has been used in remarkable ways in medicine in the past few years. One program has gotten so sophisticated at distinguishing cancerous skin lesions (such as melanomas) from benign abnormalities that it can outperform dermatologists.[7] Similar pattern recognition software is being applied to bone marrow samples to determine if machines are better at diagnosing myelodysplastic syndromes or leukemias than pathologists, or if machines can assist pathologists in making diagnoses. It's hard for me to believe any machine can outperform Karl, but this is admittedly an engrained, immutable bias of mine.

AI has already been used in assessing prognosis in myelodysplastic syndrome and has outperformed other prognostic schemas, given its ability to be applied at multiple time points in a patient's disease course.[8] In the same disease, it can predict which patients are likely to get better when treated with a particular chemotherapy, and which have cancers resistant to that chemo. If only we had known that prior to starting David on a weeks-long hospital course that was unsuccessful.

Outcomes in leukemia also should be placed in context of where we are now, two decades into the new millennium, and where we've been. In 1975, all comers with leukemia, including those with both chronic and acute varieties, had a 33 percent chance of being alive five years after a diagnosis. That survival rate has doubled, to 66 percent. With the rapidity of scientific discoveries and the incorporation of genetics and computer-based approaches accelerating as they have over the past few years, I anticipate those survival rates will increase dramatically during the next decade.

After all, the goal for me and for my clinical and research colleagues is to put ourselves out of a job as quickly as possible.

Notes

Chapter 1

1. "Welcome to Wooster: About," n.d., https://www.woosteroh.com/welcome-wooster, accessed August 14, 2018.

2. S. Perry, "Introduction to Nomenclature and Classification of Acute Leukemias," in *Nomenclature, Methodology and Results of Clinical Trials in Acute Leukemias: Recent Results in Cancer Research / Fortschritte der Krebsforschung / Progrès dans les recherches sur le cancer, vol. 43,* ed. G. Mathé, P. Pouillart, and L. Schwarzenberg (Berlin: Springer, 1973).

3. G. J. Piller, "Leukaemia—A Brief Historical Review from Ancient Times to 1950," *British Journal of Haematology* 112 (2001): 282–292; X. Thomas, "First Contributors in the History of Leukemia," *World Journal of Hematology* 2, no. 3 (2013): 62–70; J. M. Goldman and G. Q. Daley, "Chronic Myeloid Leukemia—A Brief History," in *Myeloproliferative Disorders: Hematologic Malignancies* (Berlin: Springer, 2007).

4. Cleveland Clinic, "Facts and Figures," https://my.clevelandclinic.org/about/overview/who-we-are/facts-figures, accessed August 14, 2018.

5. Source of data in table 1.1: R. L. Siegel, K. D. Miller, and A. Jemal, "Cancer Statistics, 2019," *CA Cancer Journal for Clinicians* 69

(2019): 7–34; N. Howlader, A. M. Noone, M. Krapcho, et al. (eds.), *SEER Cancer Statistics Review, 1975–2016* (Bethesda, MD: National Cancer Institute), https://seer.cancer.gov/csr/1975_2016/ (based on November 2018 SEER data submission, posted to the SEER website in April 2019); Y. Chen, H. Kantarjian, H. Wang, et al., "Acute Promyelocytic Leukemia: A Population-Based Study on Incidence and Survival in the United States, 1975–2008," *Cancer* 118, no. 23 (2012): 5811–5818.

6. T. Gilligan, "A Pathologic Fascination with Humanity," *Journal of Clinical Oncology* 36 (2017): 425–426.

7. Account of summer jobs and intern questions expanded from M. Sekeres, "How Flipping Burgers Can Cure Leukemia," *Journal of Clinical Oncology* 28 (2010): 3096–3097. Reprinted with permission, © 2010 American Society of Clinical Oncology.

8. M. A. Sekeres, J. P. Maciejewski, A. F. List, et al., "Perceptions of Disease State, Treatment Outcomes, and Prognosis among Patients with Myelodysplastic Syndromes: Results from an Internet-Based Survey," *Oncologist* 16 (2011): 904–911.

9. Regarding 7+3 treatment with cytarabine and daunorubicin, see G. Schwartsmann, A. Brondani da Rocha, R. G. Berlinck, et al., "Marine Organisms as a Source of New Anticancer Agents," *Lancet Oncology* 2 (2001): 221–225; G. Cassinelli, "The Roots of Modern Oncology: From Discovery of New Antitumor Anthracyclines to Their Clinical Use," *Tumori* 102 (2016): 226–235.

10. B. G. Arndt, J. W. Beasley, M. D. Watkinson, et al., "Tethered to the EHR: Primary Care Physician Workload Assessment Using EHR Event Log Data and Time-Motion Observations," *Annals of Family Medicine* 15, no. 5 (September 2017): 419–426.

11. For clinical studies in the late 1980s, see B. Lowenberg, R. Zittoun, H. Kerkhofs, et al., "On the Value of Intensive Remission-Induction Chemotherapy in Elderly Patients of 65+ Years with

Acute Myeloid Leukemia: A Randomized Phase III Study of the European Organization for Research and Treatment of Cancer Leukemia Group," *Journal of Clinical Oncology* 7 (1989): 1268–1274. For a "retrospective" view of supportive care, see: R. Baz, C. Rodriguez, A. Z. Fu, et al., "Impact of Remission Induction Chemotherapy on Survival in Older Adults with Acute Myeloid Leukemia," *Cancer* 110 (2007): 1752–1759.

12. *Formaldehyde, 2-Butoxyethanol and 1-tert-Butoxypropan-2-ol*, Monograph 88 (Lyon: International Agency for Research on Cancer, 2006).

Chapter 2

1. For biopsy needle, see L. A. Parapia, "Trepanning or Trephines: A History of Bone Marrow Biopsy," *British Journal of Haematology* 139 (2007): 14–19. For biopsy drill, see S. Jain, M. Enzerra, R. S. Mehta, et al., "Bone Marrow Biopsies Performed by Both the Powered OnControl Drill Device and the Jamshidi Needle Produce adequate specimens," *Journal of Clinical Pathology* 70 (2017): 541–543.

2. N. Singh Ospina, K. A. Phillips, R. Rodriguez-Gutierrez, et al., "Eliciting the Patient's Agenda-Secondary Analysis of Recorded Clinical Encounters," *Journal of General Internal Medicine* 2018, https://doi.org/10.1007/s11606-018-4540-5.

3. Stories in this section about patients' desire to understand the cause of their illness come from Mikkael A. Sekeres, "Wondering What Caused the Cancer," *New York Times*, April 21, 2016, https://well.blogs.nytimes.com/2016/04/21/wondering-what-caused-the-cancer, accessed August 15, 2018.

4. For biographical information on Sadako Sasaki, see http://sadakosasaki.com/, accessed December 10, 2018. For findings from the research on radiation and the human body, see Atomic Bomb Disease Institute, Nagasaki University, "History and Aims,"

https://www-sdc.med.nagasaki-u.ac.jp/abdi/history/index_e.html, accessed August 15, 2018; and M. Iwanaga, W. L. Hsu, M. Soda, et al., "Risk of Myelodysplastic Syndromes in People Exposed to Ionizing Radiation: A Retrospective Cohort Study of Nagasaki Atomic Bomb Survivors," *Journal of Clinical Oncology* 29 (2011): 428–434.

5. Tomas Radivoyevitch, Lynn Hlatky, Julian Landaw, et al., "Quantitative Modeling of Chronic Myeloid Leukemia: Insights from Radiobiology," *Blood* 119 (2012): 4363–4371.

6. Iwanaga et.al., "Risk of Myelodysplastic Syndromes in People Exposed to Ionizing Radiation."

7. Charlotte Jacobs, *Henry Kaplan and the Story of Hodgkin's Disease* (Stanford, CA: Stanford University Press, 2010).

8. C. Polprasert, I. Schulze, M. A. Sekeres, et al., "Inherited and Somatic Defects in DDX41 in Myeloid Neoplasms," *Cancer Cell* 27 (2015): 658–670.

9. R. Desai, D. Collett, C. J. Watson, et al., "Cancer Transmission from Organ Donors—Unavoidable but Low Risk," *Transplantation* 94 (2015): 1200–1207.

10. S. Osada, K. Horibe, K. Oiwa, et al., "A Case of Infantile Acute Monocytic Leukemia Caused by Vertical Transmission of the Mother's Leukemic Cells," *Cancer* 65 (1990): 1146–1149.

11. P. C. Nowell and D. A. Hungerford, "Chromosome Studies on Normal and Leukemic Human Leukocytes," *Journal of the National Cancer Institute* 25 (1960): 85–109.

12. J. M. Goldman and G. Q. Daley, "Chronic Myeloid Leukemia—A Brief History," in *Myeloproliferative Disorders: Hematologic Malignancies* (Berlin: Springer, 2007).

13. Ibid.

14. For an interview with Brian Druker, see C. Dreifus, "Researcher behind the Drug Gleevec," *New York Times*, November 2, 2009, https://www.nytimes.com/2009/11/03/science/03conv.html.   For an extended profile on Druker's research and Gleevec, see Terence Monmaney, "A Triumph in the War against Cancer," *Smithsonian*, May 2011, https://www.smithsonianmag.com/science-nature/a-triumph-in-the-war-against-cancer-1784705/, accessed August 19, 2019. See also, M. Deininger, E. Buchdunger, and B. J. Druker, "The Development of Imatinib as a Therapeutic Agent for Chronic Myeloid Leukemia," *Blood* 105 (2005): 2640–2653.

15. J. Druker, M. Talpaz, D. J. Resta, et al., "Efficacy and Safety of a Specific Inhibitor of the BCR-ABL Tyrosine Kinase in Chronic Myeloid Leukemia," *New England Journal of Medicine* 344 (2001): 1031–1037.

16. G. O'Brien, F. Guilhot, R. A. Larson, et al., "Imatinib Compared with Interferon and Low-Dose Cytarabine for Newly Diagnosed Chronic-Phase Chronic Myeloid Leukemia," *New England Journal of Medicine* 348 (2003): 994–1004.

17. A. Hochhaus, R. Larson, F. Guilhot, et al., "Long-Term Outcomes of Imatinib Treatment for Chronic Myeloid Leukemia," *New England Journal of Medicine* 376 (2017): 917–927; Bob Tedeschi, "The Survivors: How an Experimental Treatment Saved Patients and Changed Medicine," *StatNews*, April 25, 2017, https://www.statnews.com/2017/04/25/oncology-cancer-precision-medicine-gleevec/.

Chapter 3

1. The section on the bicycle crash first appeared in Mikkael A. Sekeres, "The Doctor Gets V.I.P. Treatment," *New York Times*, July 3, 2014, https://well.blogs.nytimes.com/2014/07/03/the-doctor-gets-vip-treatment/, accessed August 19, 2019.

2. M. A. Sekeres, P. Elson, M. E. Kalaycio, et al., "Time from Diagnosis to Treatment Initiation Predicts Survival in Younger, but Not Older, Acute Myeloid Leukemia Patients," *Blood* 113 (2009): 28–36.

3. T. C. Hoffmann and C. Del Mar, "Patients' Expectations of the Benefits and Harms of Treatments, Screening, and Tests: A Systematic Review," *Journal of the American Medical Association Internal Medicine* 175, no. 2 (2015): 274–286.

4. T. C. Hoffman and C. Del Mar, "Clinicians' Expectations of the Benefits and Harms of Treatments, Screening, and Tests," *Journal of the American Medical Association Internal Medicine* 177 (2017): 407–419.

5. Mikkael A. Sekeres, "What Our Patients Can Teach Us," *New York Times*, November 7, 2013, https://well.blogs.nytimes .com/2013/11/07/what-our-patients-can-teach-us/.

6. Mikkael A. Sekeres, "The Punishing Cost of Cancer Care," *New York Times*, December 11, 2014, https://well.blogs.nytimes .com/2014/12/11/the-punishing-cost-of-cancer-care/.

7. M. A. Sekeres, R. M. Stone, D. Zahrieh, et al., "Decision-Making and Quality of Life in Older Adults with Acute Myeloid Leukemia or Advanced Myelodysplastic Syndrome," *Leukemia* 18 (2004): 809–816.

8. S. J. Lee, F. R. Loberiza, J. D. Rizzo, et al., "Optimistic Expectations and Survival after Hematopoietic Stem Cell Transplantation," *Biology of Blood Marrow Transplant* 9 (2003): 389–396.

9. K. R. Chhabra, K. I. Pollak, S. J. Lee, et al., "Physician Communication Styles in Initial Consultations for Hematological Cancer," *Patient Education and Counseling* 93, no. 3 (2013): doi:10.1016/j .pec.2013.08.023.

10. Lee et al., "Optimistic Expectations and Survival after Hematopoietic Stem Cell Transplantation." See also International Asso-

ciation for the Study of Lung Cancer, "Lung Cancer Patients with Optimistic Attitudes Have Longer Survival, Study Finds," *ScienceDaily*, March 8, 2010, www.sciencedaily.com/releases/2010/03/100303131656.htm, accessed September 10, 2018.

11. S. J. Lee, D. Fairclough, J. H. Antin, and J. C. Weeks, "Discrepancies between Patient and Physician Estimates for the Success of Stem Cell Transplantation," *Journal of the American Medical Association* 285, no. 8 (2001): 1034–1038.

12. S. G. Thakkar, A. Z. Fu, . . . M. A. Sekeres et al., "Survival and Predictors of Outcome in Patients with Acute Leukemia Admitted to the Intensive Care Unit," *Cancer* 112, no. 10 (2008): 2233–2240.

13. L. K. Hillestad, "Acute Promyelocytic Leukemia," *Acta Medica Scandanavia* 159 (1957): 189–194.

14. L. Lo-Coco and L. Cicconi, "History of Acute Promyelocytic Leukemia: A Tale of Endless Revolution," *Mediterranean Journal of Hematology and Infectious Diseases* 3, no. 1 (2011): e2011067. doi:10.4084/MJHID.2011.067; J. D. Rowley, H. M. Golomb, and C. Dougherty, "The 15–17 Translocation: A Consistent Chromosomal Change in Acute Promyelocytic Leukaemia," *Lancet* 1, no. 8010 (March 5, 1997): 549–550.

15. J. Auer, "Some Hitherto Undescribed Structures Found in the Large Lymphocytes of a Case of Acute Leukaemia," *American Journal of the Medical Sciences* 131, no. 6 (1906): 1002–1015.

16. J. Bernard, M. Weil, M. Boiron, et al., "Acute Promyelocytic Leukaemia: Results Treatment with Daunorubicin," *Blood* 41 (1973): 489–496.

17. Z. Y. Wang and Z. Chen, "Acute Promyelocytic Leukemia: From Highly Fatal to Highly Curable," *Blood* 111 (2008): 2505–2515.

18. Ibid.

19. M. Huang, Y. Yu-Chen, C. Shu-Rong, et al., "Use of All Trans Retinoic Acid in the Treatment of Acute Promyelocytic Leukemia," *Blood* 72 (1988): 567–572.

20. Mikkael A. Sekeres, "In Sickness and in Health," *New York Times*, August 28, 2014, https://well.blogs.nytimes.com/2014/08/28/in-sickness-and-in-health.

Chapter 4

1. A. Kazi, "The Life and Times of George Washington Crile," *Journal of Postgraduate Medicine* 49, no. 3 (2003): 289–290; Ohio History Connection: Ohio History Central, Cleveland Clinic, http://www.ohiohistorycentral.org/w/Cleveland_Clinic, accessed October 12, 2018.

2. Brad Clifton, "The Cleveland Clinic X-Ray Fire of 1929," *Cleveland Historical*, https://clevelandhistorical.org/items/show/573, accessed November 12, 2018; "History of Cleveland Clinic: A Timeline," in *The Cleveland Clinic Way: Lessons in Excellence from One of the World's Leading Healthcare Organizations*, ed. T. Cosgrove (New York: McGraw-Hill, 2014), http://accessmedicine.mhmedical.com/content.aspx?bookid=2323&sectionid=180181346, accessed October 12, 2018.

3. Cleveland Clinic, "The Power of Art: The Cleveland Collection," 2017, http://www.clevelandclinic.org/lp/power-of-art, accessed August 17, 2019.

4. Cleveland Clinic, "Empathy by Design: Healing the Body While Caring for the Mind," *Washington Post*, https://www.washingtonpost.com/sf/brand-connect/cleveland-clinic/healing-while-caring-for-the-mind, accessed October 12, 2018.

5. For uses of arsenic prior and up to the 18th century, see C. Klaassen, "Heavy Metals and Heavy Metal Antagonists," in

Goodman & Gilman's The Pharmacological Basis of Therapeutics, ed. J. Hardman, A. Gilman, and L. Limbird (New York: McGraw-Hill, 1996), 1649–1672; and P. E. Bechet, "Arsenic: History of Its Use in Dermatology," *Archives of Dermatology and Syphilology* 23, no. 1 (1931): 110–117. For 19th- and 20th-century uses, see S.-X. Zhen, G.-Q. Chen, J.-H. Ni, et al., "Use of Arsenic Trioxide (As2O3) in the Treatment of Acute Promyelocytic Leukemia (APL): II. Clinical Efficacy and Pharmacokinetics in Relapsed Patients," *Blood* 89 (1997): 3354–3360.

6. For 1990s' studies of APL relapse in Shanghai, see P. Zhang, S. Y. Wang, and L. H. Hu, "Arsenic Trioxide Treated 72 Cases of Acute Promyelocytic Leukemia," *Chinese Journal of Hematology* 17 (1996): 58–62; and Zhen et al., "Use of Arsenic Trioxide (As2O3) in the Treatment of Acute Promyelocytic Leukemia (APL)." For arsenic and maturing white blood cells, see W. H. Miller Jr., H. M. Schipper, J. S. Lee, et al., "Mechanisms of Action of Arsenic Trioxide," *Cancer Research* 62 (2002): 3893–3903. For US study of relapsed APL patients, see F. Lo-Coco, and L. Cicconi, "History of Acute Promyelocytic Leukemia: A Tale of Endless Revolution," *Mediterranean Journal of Hematology and Infectious Diseases* 3(1) (2011): e2011067. doi:10.4084/MJHID.2011.067; and S. L. Soignet, S. R. Frankel, D. Douer, et al., "United States Multicenter Study of Arsenic Trioxide in Relapsed Acute Promyelocytic Leukemia," *Journal of Clinical Oncology* 19 (2001): 3852–3860.

7. A. Ghavamzadeh, K. Alimoghaddam, S. Rostami, et al., "Phase II Study of Single-Agent Arsenic Trioxide for the Front-Line Therapy of Acute Promyelocytic Leukemia," *Journal of Clinical Oncology* 29, no.20 (June 10, 2011): 2753–2757; V. Mathews, B. George, K. M. Lakshmi, et al., "Single-Agent Arsenic Trioxide in the Treatment of Newly Diagnosed Acute Promyelocytic Leukemia: Durable Remissions with Minimal Toxicity," *Blood* 107, no. 7 (April 1, 2006): 2627–2632.

8. S. L. Soignet, S. R. Frankel, D. Douer, et al., "United States Multicenter Study of Arsenic Trioxide in Relapsed Acute Promyelocytic Leukemia," *Journal of Clinical Oncology* 19 (2001): 3852–3860.

9. B. L. Powell, B. Moser, W. Stock, et al., "Arsenic Trioxide Improves Event-Free and Overall Survival for Adults with Acute Promyelocytic Leukemia: North American Leukemia Intergroup Study C9710, *Blood* 116, no. 19 (November 11, 2010): 3751–3757.

10. F. Lo-Coco, G. Avvisati, M. Vignetti, et al., "Retinoic Acid and Arsenic Ttrioxide for Acute Promyelocytic Leukemia," *New England Journal of Medicine* 369, no. 2 (July 11, 2013): 111–121.

11. Ibid.

12. Mikkael A. Sekeres, "Making Promises We Cannot Keep," *New York Times*, October 20, 2016, https://www.nytimes.com/2016/10/20/well/live/making-promises-we-cannot-keep, accessed October 20, 2018.

13. Elisabeth Kübler-Ross, *On Death and Dying* (New York: Scribner, 1969).

14. Mikkael A. Sekeres, "Seeking Calm on the Cancer Ward," *New York Times*, May 16, 2013, https://well.blogs.nytimes.com/2013/05/16/seeking-calm-on-the-cancer-ward/, accessed October 20, 2018.

15. Bob Dolgan," George Steinbrenner Left Cleveland and Became One of the Most Powerful Men in Sports," *Plain Dealer*, July 14, 2010, https://www.cleveland.com/ohio-sports-blog/index.ssf/2010/07/post_120.html, accessed October 20, 2018.

16. Mikkael A. Sekeres, "Love on the Hospital Walls," *New York Times*, December 12, 2015, http://well.blogs.nytimes.com/2015/12/17/love-on-the-hospital-walls/, accessed December 17, 2015.

17 Joan Didion, *The Year of Magical Thinking* (New York: Alfred A. Knopf, 2005).

18. M. Othus, S. Mukherjee, M. A. Sekeres, et al., "Prediction of CR Following a Second Course of '7+3' in Patients with Newly Diagnosed Acute Myeloid Leukemia not in CR after a First Course," *Leukemia* 30, no. 8 (August 2016): 1779–1780.

19. Ronald Piana, "The Evolution of U.S. Cooperative Group Trials: Publically Funded Cancer Research at a Crossroads," *American Society of Clinical Oncology Post*, March 15, 2014.

Chapter 5

1. J. P. Cohen, "The Curious Case of Gleevec Pricing," *Forbes Magazine*, https://www.forbes.com/sites/joshuacohen/2018/09/12/the-curious-case-of-gleevec-pricing/#6a48496154a3, accessed January 1, 2019; Experts in Chronic Myeloid Leukemia, "The Price of Drugs for Chronic Myeloid Leukemia (CML) Is a Reflection of the Unsustainable Prices of Cancer Drugs: From the Perspective of a Large Group of CML Experts," *Blood* 121 (2013): 4439–4442; Thomson Reuters MicroMedex Website, "AWP Policy," https://www.micromedexsolutions.com/micromedex2/4.31.0/WebHelp/RED_BOOK/AWP_Policy/AWP_Policy.htm, accessed January 2, 2019.

2. M. Herper, "Celgene, Sold for $74 Billion, Leaves a Legacy of Chutzpah in Science and Drug Pricing," *StatNews*, January 22, 2019, https://www.statnews.com/2019/01/22/celgene-legacy-chutzpah-science-drug-pricing/; S. Kaplan, "F.D.A. Names and Shames Drug Makers to Encourage Generic Competition," *New York Times*, May 18, 2018.

3. D. H. Howard, P. B. Bach, E. R. Berndt, et al., "Pricing in the Market for Anticancer Drugs," *Journal of Economic Perspectives* 29 (2015): 139–162.

4. A. Tefferi, H. Kantarjian, . . . M. A. Sekeres, et al., "In Support of a Patient-Driven Initiative and Petition to Lower the High Price of Cancer Drugs," *Mayo Clinic Proceedings* 90 (2015): 996–1000.

5. T. Neuman, J. Cubanski, J. Huang, et al., "How Much 'Skin in the Game' Is Enough? The Financial Burden of Health Spending for People in Medicare: An Updated Analysis of Out-of-Pocket Spending as a Share of Income," Henry J. Kaiser Family Foundation, June 2011, https//kaiserfamilyfoundation.files.wordpress.com/2013/01/8170.pdf.

6. S. Knoer, "What Does PBM Stand For? In Ohio (and Elsewhere), It's Programs Bilking Millions," *StatNews*, June 29, 2018, https://www.statnews.com/2018/06/29/pharmacy-benefit-managers-profits-ohio/, accessed January 2, 2019.

7. L. Noens, M. van Lierde, R. De Bock, et al., "Prevalence, Determinants, and Outcomes of Nonadherence to Imatinib Therapy in Patients with Chronic Myeloid Leukemia: The ADAGIO Study," *Blood* 113, no. 22 (2009): 5401–5411.

8. J. S. Benner, R. J. Glynn, H. Mogun, et al., "Long-term Persistence in Use of Statin Therapy in Elderly Patients," *Journal of the American Medical Association* 288, no. 4B (July 24–31, 2002): 455–461.

9. D. L. Hershman, L. H. Kushi, T. Shao, et al., "Early Discontinuation and Nonadherence to Adjuvant Hormonal Therapy in a Cohort of 8,769 Early-Stage Breast Cancer Patients," *Journal of Clinical Oncology* 28, no. 27 (September 20, 2010)): 4120–4128.

10. D. Marin, A. Bazeos, F. X. Mahon, et al., "Adherence Is the Critical Factor for Achieving Molecular Responses in Patients with Chronic Myeloid Leukemia Who Achieve Complete Cytogenetic Responses on Imatinib," *Journal of Clinical Oncology* 28, no. 14 (May 2010): 2381–2388.

11. For CML and dropping doses, see E. Jabbour, G. Saglio, J. Radich, et al., "Adherence to BCR-ABL Inhibitors: Issues for CML Therapy," *Clinical Lymphoma, Myeloma & Leukemia* 12, no. 4 (2012): 223–229. For dropping doses with AIDS, see M. A.

Chesney, J. R. Ickovics, D. B. Chambers, et al., "Self-Reported Adherence to Antiretroviral Medications among Participants in HIV Clinical Trials: The AACTG Adherence Instruments," *AIDS Care* 12 (2000): 255–266.

12. Mikkael A. Sekeres, "A Place to Be Heard," *New York Times*, December 1, 2016, https://www.nytimes.com/2016/12/01/well/live/a-place-to-be-heard.

13. National Toxicology Program, US Department of Health and Human Services, "NTP Monograph on Developmental Effects and Pregnancy Outcomes Associated with Cancer Chemotherapy Used during Cancer," May 13, 2013, http://ntp.niehs.nih.gov/ntp/ohat/cancer_chemo_preg/chemopregnancy_monofinal_508.pdf.

14. The ICU experience here expands on Mikkael A. Sekeres, "A Hallmark Moment," *Journal of Clinical Oncology* 28 (2010): 5348–5349. Reprinted with permission. ©2010 American Society of Clinical Oncology.

15. HIPAA Journal: HIPAA History, https://www.hipaajournal.com/hipaa-history/, accessed August 14, 2018.

16. P. Garfinkel, "Catering to Flyers at 30,000 Feet," *New York Times*, April 8, 2018.

17. For bacterial and fungal infections for AML patients like David, see C. Hahn-Ast, A. Glasmacher, S. Muckter, et al., "Overall Survival and Fungal Infection-Related Mortality in Patients with Invasive Fungal Infection and Neutropenia after Myelosuppressive Chemotherapy in a Tertiary Care Centre from 1995 to 2006," *Journal of Antimicrobial Chemotherapy* 65 (2010): 761–768. For APL patients see M. A. Sanz and P. Montesinos, "How We Prevent and Treat Differentiation Syndrome in Patients with Acute Promyelocytic Leukemia," *Blood* 123 (2014): 2777–2782.

18. Mikkael A. Sekeres, "Seeing God through My Patients," *New York Times*, July 9, 2015, https://well.blogs.nytimes.com/2015/07/09/seeing-god-through-my-patients/.

Chapter 6

1. M. Oken, R. Creech, D. Tormey, et al., "Toxicity and Response Criteria of the Eastern Cooperative Oncology Group," *American Journal of Clinical Oncology* 5 (1982): 649–655.

2. Source for table 6.1: D. Karnofsky and J. Burchenal, "The Clinical Evaluation of Chemotherapeutic Agents in Cancer," in *Evaluation of Chemotherapeutic Agents*, ed. C. MacLeod (New York: Columbia University Press, 1949), 191–205.

3. Source for table 6.2: "ECOG Performance Status," http://www.npcrc.org/files/news/ECOG_performance_status.pdf, as published in Oken et al., Toxicity and Response Criteria of the ECOG Group."

4. B. L. Powell, B. Moser, W. Stock, et al., "Arsenic Trioxide Improves Event-Free and Overall Survival for Adults with Acute Promyelocytic Leukemia: North American Leukemia Intergroup Study C9710," *Blood* 116, no. 19 (2010): 3751–3757.

5. Larry Hartman, "*Arsenic and Old Lace:* At the Colonial," *Harvard Crimson*, December 1, 1956, https://www.thecrimson.com/article/1956/12/1/arsenic-and-old-lace-piarsenic-and/.

6. Mikkael A. Sekeres, "Breaking Bad News to Patients," *New York Times*, September 29, 2016, https://www.nytimes.com/2016/09/29/well/live/breaking-bad-news-to-patients.

7. K. J. Norsworthy, F. Mulkey, A. F. Ward, et al., "Incidence of Differentiation Syndrome with Ivosidenib (IVO) and Enasidenib (ENA) for Treatment of Patients with Relapsed or Refractory (R/R) Isocitrate Dehydrogenase (IDH)1- or IDH2-Mutated Acute Myeloid

Leukemia (AML): A Systematic Analysis by the U.S. Food and Drug Administration (FDA)," *Blood* 132 (2018): 288a.

8. E. M. Stein, C. D. DiNardo, . . . M. A. Sekeres, et al., "Enasidenib in Mutant IDH2 Relapsed or Refractory Acute Myeloid Leukemia," *Blood* 130, no. 6 (2017): 722–731.

9. D. L. Beck, "Hazardous to Your Health: Violence in the Health-Care Workplace," *American Society of Hematology Clinical News* 4 (December 1, 2018): 134–144.

10. E. Vellenga, W. van Putten, G. J. Ossenkoppele, et al., "Autologous Peripheral Blood Stem Cell Transplantation for Acute Myeloid Leukemia," *Blood* 118 (2011): 6037–6042.

11. For the history prior to (and of) E. D. Thomas's research and procedures, see Fred Hutchinson Cancer Research Center, History of Transplantation, https://www.fredhutch.org/en/treatment/long-term-follow-up/FAQs/transplantation.html, accessed January 26, 2019; E. D. Thomas, "Bone Marrow Transplantation—Past, Present and Future," Nobel Prize lecture December 8, 1990, https://www.nobelprize.org/uploads/2018/06/thomas-lecture.pdf, accessed January 26, 2019; P. E. Rekers, M. P. Coulter, and S. Warren, "Effect of Transplantation of Bone Marrow into Irradiated Animals," *Archives of Surgery* 60 (1950): 635–667; R. B. Epstein and E. D. Thomas, "Cytogenetic Demonstration of Permanent Tolerance in Adult Outbred Dogs," *Transplantation* 5 (1967): 267–272; E. D. Thomas, G. L. Plain, T. C. Graham, et al., "Long-Term Survival of Lethally Irradiated Dogs Given Homografts of Bone Marrow," *Blood* 23 (1964): 488–493, https://ghr.nlm.nih.gov/primer/genefamily/hla, accessed January 26, 2019.

12. R. A. Gatti, H. J. Meuwissen, H. D. Allen, et al., "Immunological Reconstitution of Sex-Linked Lymphopenic Immunological Deficiency," *Lancet* 2 (1969): 1366–1369.

13. R. L. Powles, G. R. Morgenstern, and H. E. Kay, "Mismatched Family Donors for Bone-Marrow Transplantation as Treatment for Acute Leukaemia," *Lancet* 1 (1983): 612–615.

14. Gatti et al., "Immunological Reconstitution of Sex-Linked Lymphopenic Immunological Deficiency."

15. E. Gluckman, H. E. Broxmeyer, A. D. Auerbach, et al., "Hematopoietic Reconstitution in a Patient with Fanconi's Anemia by Means of Umbilical Cord Blood from an HLA-Identical Sibling," *New England Journal of Medicine* 321 (1989): 1174–1178; E. Gluckman, "History of Cord Blood Transplantation," *Bone Marrow Transplantation* 44 (2009): 621–626; K. K. Ballen and T. R. Spitzer, "The Great Debate: Haploidentical or Cord Blood Transplant," *Bone Marrow Transplantation* 46 (2011): 323–329.

16. A. D'Souza and C. Fretham, "Current Uses and Outcomes of Hematopoietic Cell Transplantation (HCT): CIBMTR Summary Slides," 2017, available at http://www.cibmtr.org, accessed January 26, 2019.

17. Be The Match, "How Does a Patient's Ethnic Background Affect Matching?" https://bethematch.org/transplant-basics/matching-patients-with-donors/how-does-a-patients-ethnic-background-affect-matching/, accessed January 26, 2019.

18. M. A. Bellis, K. Hughes, S. Hughes, et al., "Measuring Paternal Discrepancy and Its Public Health Consequences," *Journal of Epidemiology & Community Health* 59 (2005): 749–754; R. W. Marsters, "Determination of Nonpaternity by Blood Groups," *Journal of Forensic Science* 2 (1957): 15–37.

19. P. Rincon, "Study Debunks Illegitimacy 'Myth,'" BBC News, February 11, 2009, http://news.bbc.co.uk/2/hi/science/nature/7881652.stm, accessed January 16, 2019.

20. D. W. Soderdahl, D. Rabah, T. McCune, et al., "Misattributed Paternity in a Living Related Donor: To Disclose or Not to

Disclose?" *Urology* 64 (2004): 590; A. Young, S. Kim, E. Gibney, et al., "Discovering Misattributed Paternity in Living Kidney Donation: Prevalence, Preference, and Practice," *Transplantation* 87 (2009): 1429–1435.

21. L. Ross, "Good Ethics Requires Good Science: Why Transplant Programs Should Not Disclose Misattributed Parentage," *American Journal of Transplantation* 10 (2010): 742–746.

22. S. Jacobson, J. Eggert, J. Deluca, et al., "Misattributed Paternity in Hematopoietic Stem Cell Transplantation: The Role of the Healthcare Provider," *Clinical Journal of Oncology Nursing* 19 (2015): 218–221.

23. R. Green, J. Berg, W. Grody, et al., "ACMG Recommendation for Reporting of Incidental Findings in Clinical Exome and Genome Sequencing," *Genetics in Medicine* 15 (2013): 565–574.

Chapter 7

1. R. Kronenberger, E. Schleyer, M. Bornhauser, et al., "Imatinib in Breast Milk," *Annals of Hematology* 88 (2009): 1265–1266.

2. For lab test, see R. Saiki, D. Gelfand, S. Stoffel, et al., "Primer-Directed Enzymatic Amplification of DNA with a Thermostable DNA Polymerase," *Science* 239 (1988): 487–491. See also K. B. Mullis, "The Polymerase Chain Reaction," Nobel Lecture, December 8, 1993, https://www.nobelprize.org/prizes/chemistry/1993/mullis/lecture/, accessed February 18, 2019.

3. T. P. Hughes, J. Kaeda, S. Branford, et al., "Frequency of Major Molecular Responses to Imatinib or Interferon Alfa Plus Cytarabine in Newly Diagnosed Chronic Myeloid Leukemia," *New England Journal of Medicine* 349 (2003): 1423–1432.

4. D. Marin, A. R. Ibrahim, C. Lucas, et al., "Assessment of BCR-ABL1 Transcript Levels at 3 Months Is the Only Requirement for

Predicting Outcome for Patients with Chronic Myeloid Leukemia Treated with Tyrosine Kinase Inhibitors," *Journal of Clinical Oncology* 30 (2011): 232–238.

5. G. Saglio, D. W. Kim, S. Issaragrisil, et al., "Nilotinib versus Imatinib for Newly Diagnosed Chronic Myeloid Leukemia," *New England Journal of Medicine* 362 (2010): 2251–2259; H. Kantarjian, N. P. Shah, A. Hochhaus, et al., "Dasatinib versus Imatinib in Newly Diagnosed Chronic-Phase Chronic Myeloid Leukemia," *New England Journal of Medicine* 362 (2010): 2260–2270.

6. J. E. Cortes, G. Saglio, H. M. Kantarjian, et al., "Final 5-Year Study Results of DASISION: The Dasatinib versus Imatinib Study in Treatment-Naïve Chronic Myeloid Leukemia Patients Trial," *Journal of Clinical Oncology* 34, no. 20 (July 10, 2016): 2333–2340. A. Hochhaus, G. Saglio, T. P. Hughes, et al., "Long-Term Benefits and Risks of Frontline Nilotinib vs. Imatinib for Chronic Myeloid Leukemia in Chronic Phase: 5-Year Update of the Randomized ENESTnd Trial," *Leukemia* 30 (2016): 1044–1054.

7. Americord: Compare Cord Blood Banks, https://compare .americordblood.com/comparecordbloodcosts/results, accessed February 24, 2019.

8. J. J. Nietfeld, M. C. Pasquini, B. R. Logan, et al., "Lifetime Probabilities of Hematopoietic Stem Cell Transplantation in the U.S.," *Biology of Blood Marrow Transplantation* 14, no. 3 (2008): 316–322.

9. National Geographic, "Flash Facts about Lightning," June 24, 2005, https://news.nationalgeographic.com/news/2004/06/flash -facts-about-lightning/, accessed February 24, 2019.

10. A. M. Noone, N. Howlader, M. Krapcho, et al., eds., *SEER Cancer Statistics Review,* 1975–2015, National Cancer Institute, Bethesda, MD, https://seer.cancer.gov/csr/1975_2015/, based on November 2017 SEERHdata submission, posted to the SEER

website, April 2018. For leukemia stats, see https://seer.cancer.gov/archive/csr/1975_2015/results_merged/sect_13_leukemia.pdf, accessed August 18, 2019.

11. K. B. Gale, A. M. Ford, R. Repp, et al., "Backtracking Leukemia to Birth: Identification of Clonotypic Gene Fusion Sequences in Neonatal Blood Spots," *Proceeding of the National Academy of Sciences of the USA* 94, no. 25 (1997): 13950–13954.

12. Jason Gonzalez, Monte S. Willis, and Robert Guthrie, "Clinical Chemistry/Microbiology," *Laboratory Medicine* 40, no. 12 (December 1, 2009): 748–749.

13. J. L. Wiemels, G. Cazzaniga, M. Daniotti, et al., "Prenatal Origin of Acute Lymphoblastic Leukaemia in Children," *Lancet* 354 (1999): 1499–1503.

14. D. M. Ross, S. Branford, J. F. Seymour, et al., "Safety and Efficacy of Imatinib Cessation for CML Patients with Stable Undetectable Minimal Residual Disease: Results from the TWISTER Study," *Blood* 22, no. 4 (July 25, 2013): 515–522; F. X. Mahon, D. Réa, J. Guilhot, et al., "Discontinuation of Imatinib in Patients with Chronic Myeloid Leukaemia Who Have Maintained Complete Molecular Rremission for at Least 2 Years: The Prospective, Multicentre Stop Imatinib (STIM) Trial," *Lancet Oncology* 11, no. 11 (November 2010): 1029–1035.

15. S. Saussele, J. Richter, J. Guilhot, et al., "Discontinuation of Tyrosine Kinase Inhibitor Therapy in Chronic Myeloid Leukaemia (EURO-SKI): A Prespecified Interim Analysis of a Prospective, Multicentre, Non-Randomised, Trial," *Lancet Oncology* 19, no. 6 (June 2018): 747–757.

16. ESPN.com News Services, "Friday's Game Called 1 Strike Away from Being Official," http://www.espn.com/mlb/news/story?id=2828833, accessed March 10, 2019.

17. T. W. LeBlanc and M. R. Litzow, "Are Transfusions a Barrier to High-Quality End-of-Life Care in Hematology?" *Hematologist* 15 (2018): 13.

18. For survey of 350 specialists, see O. O. Odejide, A. M. Cronin, C. C. Earle, et al., "Why Are Patients with Blood Cancers More Likely to Die without Hospice?" *Cancer* 123 (2017): 3377–3384. For SEER analysis, see S. A. Fletcher, A. M. Cronin, A. M. Zeidan, et al., "Intensity of End-of-Life Care for Patients with Myelodysplastic Syndromes: Findings from a Large National Database," *Cancer* 122 (2016): 1209–1215. For patients dependent on transfusions, see A. J. Olszewski, P. C. Egan, and T. W. LeBlanc, "Transfusion Dependence and Use of Hospice among Medicare Beneficiaries with Leukemia," *Blood* 130 (2017): 277.

19. J. R. Lowe, Y. Yu, S. Wolf, et al., "A Cohort Study of Patient-Reported Outcomes and Healthcare Utilization in Acute Myeloid Leukemia Patients Receiving Active Cancer Therapy in the Last Six Months of Life," *Journal of Palliative Medicine* 21 (2018): 592–597.

20. Mikkael A. Sekeres, "A Patient's Goal: Get Him to the Church on Time," *New York Times*, December 6, 2012, https://well .blogs.nytimes.com/2012/12/06/a-wedding-and-a-funeral/, accessed March 10, 2019.

21. D. C. Young and E. M. Hade, "Holidays, Birthdays, and Postponement of Cancer Death," *Journal of the American Medical Association* 292 (2004): 3012–3016.

22. ESPN.com News Services, "Fan Wants Browns Pallbearers," July 9, 2013, http://www.espn.com/nfl/story/_/id/9459655/cleveland -browns-fan-takes-last-shot-team-obituary, accessed March 10, 2019.

23. J. Canaani, B. N. Savani, M. Labopin, et al., "Donor Age Determines Outcome in Acute Leukemia Patients over 40 Undergoing

Haploidentical Hematopoietic Cell Transplantation," *American Journal of Hematology* 93 (2018): 246–253.

24. American Cancer Society, "What's It Like to Get a Stem Cell Transplant?" https://www.cancer.org/treatment/treatments-and -side-effects/treatment-types/stem-cell-transplant/process.html, accessed March 10, 2019.

Epilogue

1. Mikkael A. Sekeres, "Cured from Cancer, Almost," *New York Times*, May 11, 2015, https://well.blogs.nytimes.com/2015/05/11/ cured-from-cancer-almost/, accessed March 20, 2019.

2. R. M. Stone, S. J. Mandrekar, B. L. Sanford, et al., "Midostau-rin plus Chemotherapy for Acute Myeloid Leukemia with a FLT3 Mutation," *New England Journal of Medicine* 377, no. 5 (August 3, 2017): 454–464; "FDA Approves Gilteritinib for Relapsed or Refractory Acute Myeloid Leukemia (fGonzalAML) with a FLT3 Mutation," https://www.fda.gov/Drugs/InformationOnDrugs/ ApprovedDrugs/ucm627045.htm.

3. E. M. Stein, C. D. DiNardo, . . . M. A. Sekeres, et al., "Enasidenib in Mutant-*IDH2* Relapsed or Refractory Acute Myeloid Leukemia," *Blood* 130, no. 6 (August 10, 2017): 722–731; C. D. DiNardo, E. M. Stein, . . . M. A. Sekeres, et al., "Durable Remissions with Ivo-sidenib in IDH1-Mutated Relapsed or Refractory AML," *New England Journal of Medicine,* 378, no. 25 (June 21, 2017): 2386–2398.

4. David A. Sallman, Amy DeZern, Kendra Sweet, et al., "Phase Ib/II Combination Study of APR-246 and Azacitidine (AZA) in Patients with *TP53* Mutant Myelodysplastic Syndromes (MDS) and Acute Myeloid Leukemia (AML)" (abstract), in *Proceedings of the American Association for Cancer Research Annual Meeting 2018,* April 14–18, 2018, Chicago (IL), Philadelphia (PA): AACR; *Cancer Research* 78, Suppl. 3 (2018): abstract no. CT068.

5. J. H. Park, I. Rivière, M. Gonen, et al., "Long-Term Follow-up of CD19 CAR Therapy in Acute Lymphoblastic Leukemia," *New England Journal of Medicine* 378, no. 5 (February 1, 2018): 449–459.

6. P. Jain, H. Kantarjian, P. C. Boddu, et al., "Analysis of Cardiovascular and Arteriothrombotic Adverse Events in Chronic-Phase CML Patients after Frontline TKIs," *Blood Advances* 3, no. 6 (2019): 851–861.

7. H. A. Haenssle, C. Fink, R. Schneiderbauer, et al., "Man against Machine: Diagnostic Performance of a Deep Learning Convolutional Neural Network for Dermoscopic Melanoma Recognition in Comparison to 58 Dermatologists," *Annals of Oncology* 29, no. 8 (August 1, 2018): 1836–1842.

8. A. Nazha, R. S. Komrokji, . . . M. A. Sekeres, et al., "A Personalized Prediction Model to Risk Stratify Patients with Myelodysplastic Syndromes," *Blood* 132, Suppl. 1 (2018): 793, https://seer.cancer.gov/statfacts/html/leuks.html, accessed March 10, 2019.

Index